Optimizing the Process for Establishing the *Dietary Guidelines for Americans*

THE SELECTION PROCESS

Committee to Review the Process to Update the *Dietary Guidelines for Americans*

Food and Nutrition Board

Health and Medicine Division

A Consensus Study Report of

The National Academies of
SCIENCES · ENGINEERING · MEDICINE

THE NATIONAL ACADEMIES PRESS
Washington, DC
www.nap.edu

THE NATIONAL ACADEMIES PRESS 500 Fifth Street, NW Washington, DC 20001

This activity was supported by Contract No. AG-3198-C-16-0004 from the U.S. Department of Agriculture. Any opinions, findings, conclusions, or recommendations expressed in this publication do not necessarily reflect the views of any organization or agency that provided support for the project.

International Standard Book Number-13: 978-0-309-45360-8
International Standard Book Number-10: 0-309-45360-7
Digital Object Identifier: https://doi.org/10.17226/24637

Additional copies of this publication are available for sale from the National Academies Press, 500 Fifth Street, NW, Keck 360, Washington, DC 20001; (800) 624-6242 or (202) 334-3313; http://www.nap.edu.

Printed in the United States of America

Suggested citation: National Academies of Sciences, Engineering, and Medicine. 2017. *Optimizing the process for establishing the* Dietary Guidelines for Americans: *The selection process*. Washington, DC: The National Academies Press. doi: https://doi.org/10.17226/24637.

The National Academies of
SCIENCES • ENGINEERING • MEDICINE

The **National Academy of Sciences** was established in 1863 by an Act of Congress, signed by President Lincoln, as a private, nongovernmental institution to advise the nation on issues related to science and technology. Members are elected by their peers for outstanding contributions to research. Dr. Marcia McNutt is president.

The **National Academy of Engineering** was established in 1964 under the charter of the National Academy of Sciences to bring the practices of engineering to advising the nation. Members are elected by their peers for extraordinary contributions to engineering. Dr. C. D. Mote, Jr., is president.

The **National Academy of Medicine** (formerly the Institute of Medicine) was established in 1970 under the charter of the National Academy of Sciences to advise the nation on medical and health issues. Members are elected by their peers for distinguished contributions to medicine and health. Dr. Victor J. Dzau is president.

The three Academies work together as the **National Academies of Sciences, Engineering, and Medicine** to provide independent, objective analysis and advice to the nation and conduct other activities to solve complex problems and inform public policy decisions. The National Academies also encourage education and research, recognize outstanding contributions to knowledge, and increase public understanding in matters of science, engineering, and medicine.

Learn more about the National Academies of Sciences, Engineering, and Medicine at **www.nationalacademies.org.**

The National Academies of

SCIENCES · ENGINEERING · MEDICINE

Consensus Study Reports published by the National Academies of Sciences, Engineering, and Medicine document the evidence-based consensus on the study's statement of task by an authoring committee of experts. Reports typically include findings, conclusions, and recommendations based on information gathered by the committee and the committee's deliberations. Each report has been subjected to a rigorous and independent peer-review process and it represents the position of the National Academies on the statement of task.

Proceedings published by the National Academies of Sciences, Engineering, and Medicine chronicle the presentations and discussions at a workshop, symposium, or other event convened by the National Academies. The statements and opinions contained in proceedings are those of the participants and are not endorsed by other participants, the planning committee, or the National Academies.

For information about other products and activities of the National Academies, please visit www.nationalacademies.org/about/whatwedo.

COMMITTEE TO REVIEW THE PROCESS TO UPDATE THE *DIETARY GUIDELINES FOR AMERICANS*

ROBERT M. RUSSELL (*Chair*), Professor Emeritus, Nutrition and Medicine, Tufts University School of Medicine, Boston, MA

JAMY ARD, Professor, Department of Epidemiology and Prevention; Co-Director, Wake Forest Baptist Health Weight Management Center, Wake Forest University Baptist Medical Center, Winston-Salem, NC

STEPHANIE A. ATKINSON, Professor, Pediatrics, McMaster University, Hamilton, ON

CAROL J. BOUSHEY, Associate Researcher, Professor, Cancer Epidemiology Program; Director, Nutrition Support Shared Resource, University of Hawaii Cancer Center, Honolulu

SUSAN M. KREBS-SMITH, Chief, Risk Factor Assessment Branch, Epidemiology and Genomics Research Program, Division of Cancer Control and Population Sciences, National Cancer Institute, Bethesda, MD

JOSEPH LAU, Professor Emeritus, Center for Evidence Synthesis in Health, Department of Health Services, Policy & Practice, Brown University School of Public Health, Providence, RI

BRUCE Y. LEE, Director, Operations Research, International Vaccine Access Center; Executive Director, Global Obesity Prevention Center; Associate Professor, International Health, Johns Hopkins Bloomberg School of Public Health, Baltimore, MD

JOANNE R. LUPTON, Distinguished Professor Emerita, Texas A&M University, College Station

SALLY C. MORTON, Dean, College of Science, Virginia Tech, Blacksburg

NICOLAAS P. PRONK, President, HealthPartners Institute; Chief Science Officer, HealthPartners, Minneapolis, MN

SUSAN B. ROBERTS, Director, Energy Metabolism Laboratory and Professor of Nutrition, U.S. Department of Agriculture Human Nutrition Research Center on Aging at Tufts University; Professor of Psychiatry and Staff Member in Pediatrics, Tufts Medical School, Boston, MA

A. CATHARINE ROSS, Professor, Nutrition and Physiology; Dorothy Foehr Chair and Professor, Department of Nutritional Sciences, The Pennsylvania State University, University Park

---

NOTE: See Appendix D, Disclosure of Conflicts of Interest.

BARBARA O. SCHNEEMAN, Emeritus Professor of Nutrition, Department of Nutrition and Department of Food Science and Technology, University of California, Davis
MARTÍN J. SEPÚLVEDA, IBM Fellow, Retired IBM Vice President of Health Systems and Policy Research, Watson Research Laboratory, IBM Corporation, St. Augustine, FL

Health and Medicine Division Study Staff

SAMANTHA M. CHAO, Study Director
MEGHAN E. QUIRK, Senior Program Officer
ANNA BURY, Research Associate
MEREDITH J. YOUNG, Senior Program Assistant
ANN L. YAKTINE, Director, Food and Nutrition Board

Reviewers

This Consensus Study Report was reviewed in draft form by individuals chosen for their diverse perspectives and technical expertise. The purpose of this independent review is to provide candid and critical comments that will assist the National Academies of Sciences, Engineering, and Medicine in making each published report as sound as possible and to ensure that it meets the institutional standards for quality, objectivity, evidence, and responsiveness to the study charge. The review comments and draft manuscript remain confidential to protect the integrity of the deliberative process.

We thank the following individuals for their review of this report:

DAVID B. ALLISON, University of Alabama at Birmingham
KIRSTEN BIBBINS-DOMINGO, University of California, San Francisco
NANCY F. BUTTE, Baylor College of Medicine
CHRISTINA ECONOMOS, Tufts University
PHILIP GLEASON, Mathematica Policy Research, Inc.
PETER BARTON HUTT, Covington & Burling, LLP
EILEEN KENNEDY, Tufts University
RONALD KRAUSS, Children's Hospital Oakland Research Institute
PENNY KRIS-ETHERTON, The Pennsylvania State University
SYDNE JENNIFER NEWBERRY, RAND Corporation
CHRISTOPHER H. SCHMID, Brown University

ALISON STEIBER, Academy of Nutrition and Dietetics
PATRICK J. STOVER, Cornell University

Although the reviewers listed above provided many constructive comments and suggestions, they were not asked to endorse the conclusions or recommendations of this report nor did they see the final draft before its release. The review of this report was overseen by **DIANE F. BIRT** of Iowa State University and **JOHANNA T. DWYER** of Tufts Medical Center. They were responsible for making certain that an independent examination of this report was carried out in accordance with the standards of the National Academies and that all review comments were carefully considered. Responsibility for the final content rests entirely with the authoring committee and the National Academies.

Preface

Federal guidance on nutrition and diet is published every 5 years in a document called the *Dietary Guidelines for Americans* (*DGA*). This publication is intended to provide up-to-date nutrition information for the U.S. public and has become the basis for federal nutrition policies and programs. However, Congress has recently questioned whether the processes whereby this guidance is developed, interpreted, and disseminated are optimal and balanced, and now has mandated a comprehensive review of the entire process.

This Consensus Study Report is a product of a special ad hoc committee that was appointed by the National Academies of Sciences, Engineering, and Medicine (the National Academies) to review the processes for each of the following:

1. How the selection process for the Dietary Guidelines Advisory Committee (DGAC) can be improved to provide more transparency, eliminate bias, and include committee members with a range of viewpoints;
2. How the Nutrition Evidence Library (NEL) is compiled and used, including whether the NEL reviews and other systematic reviews and data analysis are conducted according to rigorous and objective scientific standards;
3. How systematic reviews are conducted on long-standing DGAC recommendations, including whether scientific studies are included from scientists with a range of viewpoints; and
4. How the *DGA* can better prevent chronic disease, ensure nutritional sufficiency for all Americans, and accommodate a range of individual factors, including age, gender, and metabolic health.

This present report is the first of two reports by this committee. This first short report reviews data and makes recommendations pertinent to question 1 (above) *only*: the selection process. A second report will later review data and make recommendations pertaining to questions 2–4.

Although our National Academies committee grounded its work in as much evidence as possible, there are scanty data available on how best to judge the effectiveness of a selection process for populating a committee such as the DGAC. Thus, reasoning and informed judgment were often used by our committee in making its recommendations that would serve to enhance transparency, balance, and inclusiveness—while minimizing undue influences—in the DGAC selection process. The reasoning used by our committee is fully described in Chapter 4 of this report.

The *DGA* is a report of national significance in that it serves as the basis for all federal nutrition policies and federal nutrition assistance programs. The scientific report of the DGAC itself provides nutritional and dietary information to the public for the intended purpose of promoting health and preventing disease. Thus, the process for getting to a final *DGA* report is necessarily a long, complicated, and iterative one. Our committee had to struggle in limiting the scope of our meetings to the selection process only, as the DGAC selection process itself could have implications for the rest of the processes used for updating the *DGA*. For example, if specific topics were to be chosen as main foci for an update to the *DGA*, this could influence the DGAC's composition. The opposite could also be true—the persons selected for a DGAC might readily influence the guidelines chosen for emphasis in updating. Due to the 4-month time constraint that our committee was under for issuing our report on the selection process, several such interrelated issues could not be fully explored. These issues, however, will be more fully addressed in our second report. Nevertheless, the recommendations we make in this report should stand, regardless of any considerations encountered for answering questions 2–4 in our second report.

This committee for addressing DGAC process improvement wishes to sincerely thank the many experts who assisted us with this first report by giving presentations, written commentary, and other means. And, of course, special thanks are owed to the U.S. Department of Agriculture, the sponsor of this report, and to the staff of the Food and Nutrition Board of the Health and Medicine Division of the National Academies led by Samantha Chao. It does not need to be said that it is because of the staff that most of the work is done and the task gets completed on time.

Robert M. Russell, *Chair*
Committee to Review the Process to Update the
Dietary Guidelines for Americans

Acknowledgments

The committee and staff would like to thank those who presented statements and presentations at the public workshops held on September 1, 2016, via WebEx, and on October 17, 2016, in Washington, DC:

Richard Black, Quadrant D Consulting
Kellie Casavale, U.S. Department of Health and Human Services (HHS)
Sheldon Greenfield, University of California, Irvine
Peter Jacobson, University of Michigan
Quyen Ngo-Metzger, Agency for Healthcare Research and Quality
Julie Obbagy, U.S. Department of Agriculture (USDA)
Eve Essery Stoody, USDA
Angela Tagtow, USDA
Walter Willett, Harvard University

We would like to thank those who provided oral and written public comment to the committee. We would also like to thank the General Services Administration for its helpful background information. In addition, there are many National Academies of Sciences, Engineering, and Medicine staff members who helped throughout the study process. The staff would like to thank Clyde Behney, Peter Blair, Mattie Cohan, Chelsea Frakes, Renee Gethers, Faye Hillman, Jim Hinchman, Sarah Kelley, Rose Marie Martinez, and Tina Ritter. Finally, we would like to thank and recognize USDA for sponsoring this study and for its helpful background information.

Contents

SUMMARY 1

1 INTRODUCTION 13

The *Dietary Guidelines for Americans*, 14

Evaluation by the National Academies of Sciences, Engineering, and Medicine, 18

References, 21

2 THE DIETARY GUIDELINES ADVISORY COMMITTEE PROCESS 23

A Brief History, 23

Establishment of a Federal Advisory Committee, 24

Current Advisory Committee Selection Process, 32

Dietary Guidelines Advisory Committee Operating Process, 34

Conclusion, 35

References, 35

3 MODELS FOR COMPOSING AN ADVISORY COMMITTEE 37

Various Selection Processes Used for Federal Advisory Committees, 38

Selection Processes Used for Non-FACA Committees, 55

Conclusion, 59

References, 60

4 OPPORTUNITIES TO BUILD TRUST **65**
Assessment of the DGAC Selection Process, 65
Enhance Transparency During Candidate Review, 68
Criteria for Selecting Candidates, 73
DGAC Composition, 75
Additional Public Comment Periods, 77
Addressing Biases and Conflicts of Interest, 80
Conclusion, 87
References, 87

5 A CONTINUOUSLY LEARNING SELECTION PROCESS **91**
A Vision for Continuous Quality Improvement, 91
Application to the DGAC Selection Process, 92
Conclusion, 96
References, 96

APPENDIXES

A LITERATURE SEARCH STRATEGY FOR "CONFLICT OF INTEREST" 99
B PUBLIC WORKSHOP AGENDAS AND COMMENTS 105
C COMMITTEE MEMBER AND STAFF BIOGRAPHIES 109
D DISCLOSURE OF CONFLICTS OF INTEREST 121

Summary[1]

Federal guidance on nutrition and diet is intended to reflect the state of the science and deliver the most reliable recommendations possible according to the best available evidence. This guidance, updated and presented every 5 years in the *Dietary Guidelines for Americans* (*DGA*), serves as the basis for all federal nutrition policies and nutrition assistance programs, as well as nutrition education programs. Despite the use of the guidelines over the past 30 years, recent challenges prompted Congress to question the process by which food and nutrition guidance is developed.

The *DGA* is a report that provides nutritional and dietary information to the public for the purpose of promoting health and preventing disease. To help Americans make healthy food choices, the U.S. Department of Agriculture (USDA) and the U.S. Department of Health and Human Services (HHS) are mandated by Congress in the National Nutritional Monitoring and Related Research Act of 1990 to jointly review and author the guidelines through a multistep process to reflect "the preponderance of the scientific and medical knowledge which is current at the time the report is prepared." The process to create the guidelines is not simple, and it changes as the science evolves. The process begins with an assessment of relevant scientific data by a federal advisory committee selected and convened by USDA and HHS. This panel of nationally recognized experts, known as the Dietary Guidelines Advisory Committee (DGAC), indepen-

[1]This summary does not include references. Citations for the findings presented in the summary appear in subsequent chapters of the report.

dently evaluates the scientific evidence and makes recommendations to the departments about how the *DGA* could be revised. The conclusions of the DGAC are submitted to the secretaries of USDA and HHS in the form of a scientific report and are only advisory; they do not constitute draft policy. The DGAC report serves as the scientific basis for the next edition of the *DGA*.

When the 2015 DGAC released its report, some of the content received criticism from different stakeholders leading to questions about the advisory committee's composition and membership selection processes. Further questions were raised about the breadth of the DGAC's scope, the processes used to evaluate the evidence, and the completeness of the advisory committee's work.

CHARGE TO THE NATIONAL ACADEMIES OF SCIENCES, ENGINEERING, AND MEDICINE

In response to concerns raised about the *2015–2020 DGA*, Congress mandated that the National Academies of Sciences, Engineering, and Medicine (the National Academies) evaluate the entire process used to develop the *DGA*. Specifically, the Consolidated Appropriations Act, 2016, calls for a review of the following:

1. How the advisory committee selection process can be improved to provide more transparency, eliminate bias, and include committee members with a range of viewpoints;
2. How the Nutrition Evidence Library (NEL) is compiled and utilized, including whether NEL reviews and other systematic reviews and data analysis are conducted according to rigorous and objective scientific standards;
3. How systematic reviews are conducted on long-standing *DGA* recommendations, including whether scientific studies are included from scientists with a range of viewpoints; and
4. How the *DGA* can better prevent chronic disease, ensure nutritional sufficiency for all Americans, and accommodate a range of individual factors, including age, gender, and metabolic health.

The National Academies appointed 14 members to the Committee to Review the Process to Update the *Dietary Guidelines for Americans*. Specifically, the task is to assess the process used to develop the guidelines, and not evaluate the substance or use of the guidelines (see Chapter 1 for the full statement of task). The committee was asked to respond to the first part of the task: "How the advisory committee selection process can be improved to provide more transparency, eliminate bias, and include committee members with a range of viewpoints," in a first short report for the purpose of informing the 2020 cycle, which is scheduled to begin in early 2017. As part of an overall, comprehensive review of the process to update the *DGA*, additional findings and recommendations about the selection process may be made as part of this committee's next report.

MODELS FOR COMPOSING AN ADVISORY COMMITTEE

The DGAC is established in pursuit of fulfilling the National Nutrition Monitoring and Related Research Act and governed by the Federal Advisory Committee Act (FACA), which directs the establishment, operation, oversight, and termination of advisory committees within the executive branch of the federal government. To comply with FACA, a number of administrative processes must be followed to institute each DGAC, including filing a charter and developing a plan to fairly balance membership.[2] Other administrative tasks used by USDA and HHS include updating bylaws, updating the charge, and preparing a database for public comments. Once the federal advisory committee is established, steps used by USDA and HHS for selecting members include soliciting candidates, reviewing nomination packages and creating a slate of potential members, approving the slate, and finally, formal appointment.

This National Academies committee sought to ground its work in as much evidence as possible but found few objective measures to assess the effectiveness of a selection process. An exploratory search of other advisory committees' selection processes—including those that are and are not governed by FACA—identified a number of differing noteworthy models. This search revealed a lack of standardization for how experts are nominated, screened, vetted, and appointed to a committee. No set of best practices to promote transparency and engage a broad set of viewpoints and expertise could be identified. Although there are certain similarities in the selection processes used by federal advisory committees, wide variations exist in how the selection of advisory committees is operationalized. Additionally, some advisory committees make use of stakeholder representatives with varying levels of involvement, while others only engage stakeholder groups through public comments. Identified differences alluded to each advisory committee's unique origins and goals.

One important difference identified among advisory committees is the approaches used to address biases and conflicts of interest. For the purpose of selecting members to the DGAC, it is important to interpret

[2]The administrative lead department switches between USDA and HHS every 5 years. The department with the lead is responsible for following the appropriate processes.

conflicts of interest broadly by including not only financial sources, but also *nonfinancial* conflicts of interest (e.g., statements in publications, history of unpaid advisory roles, organizational affiliations). Defined this broadly, it might not always be possible to entirely eliminate biases and conflicts of interest on a panel of experts. The ultimate goal of limiting and managing conflicts of interest is to develop a trustworthy process and create reliable guidelines, independent from undue influences. Significant conflicts ought to be avoided, but some situations may exist where the requisite expertise cannot be found in individuals without some conflicts of interest. In these instances, it is necessary to identify, disclose, and manage the influences in question.

OPPORTUNITIES TO BUILD TRUST

The goal of this review is to provide recommendations to develop a trustworthy process for creating the *DGA*. One critical but early step that can be taken to ensure the *DGA* is reliable is to optimize the integrity of the selection process. This National Academies committee identified a set of values to enhance the integrity of the selection process:

1. *Enhance transparency.* To the extent practicable, each step ought to be described in as much detail as possible and be made available to the public for its understanding. This transparency can help reassure the public that no undue influences or untoward actions are being taken.
2. *Promote diversity of expertise and experience.* A broad range of expertise and experience must be considered to create a balanced committee. Expertise has to align with the topic areas to be reviewed. Diversity with respect to nontechnical skills (e.g., ability to form consensus or develop compromise) also needs to be considered. Building on the first characteristic of transparency, involvement from a broad range of perspectives, including public involvement, is also critical to fostering diversity.
3. *Support a deliberative process.* A deliberative process should be used that considers information from a wide variety of sources. Decision makers ought to freely exchange information with one another toward the goal of coming to agreement or consensus. To the extent possible, the public should be engaged as well.
4. *Manage biases and conflicts of interest.* The biases of individual members should be balanced among a broad representation of perspectives. Actual and/or perceived conflicts of interest—both financial and nonfinancial—should be eliminated to the extent possible or their effects be minimized.

5. *Adopt state-of-the-art processes and methods.* As practicable, selection processes and actions ought to be based on the best available evidence for the broader purpose of managing bias and conflict of interest. They should be revised and improved on as new evidence arises.

This National Academies committee compared these values of an "ideal" selection process to the current DGAC selection process. The committee found that, overall, the DGAC selection process is thoughtful and works within the bounds of the relevant laws to serve USDA and HHS, as well as the American public. However, the lack of transparency in the current process could lead to the perception that the membership of the DGAC is inequitable, which affects its integrity and trustworthiness. Specifically, the step currently used to "conduct a review of nominations and propose a slate of candidates" was found to be largely subjective and could be improved. The other steps were generally more direct and were not deemed to inhibit trust. Recommendations and suggestions are offered specifically in response to this step to enhance transparency and inclusiveness, and minimize undue influences (see Figure S-1).

Review of Candidates

"Conduct a review of nominations and propose a slate of candidates," step 3 of the current process, is inherently the most subjective step in the DGAC selection process. Concern has been expressed that the departments are not fairly considering all qualified candidates and not including members with a broad spectrum of perspectives. Unfortunately, there are limited objective measures to judge a nominee's qualifications and the overall balance of a committee.

A more transparent process to review candidates is needed, as the mandate from Congress indicates that some subsets of the public do not trust the *DGA*. Based on lessons learned from an evaluation of other advisory committees, this National Academies committee concludes that the initial screening of nominees should be separated from the appointment authority. A neutral, unbiased arbiter should evaluate candidates' nomination packages and qualifications, identify other candidates as necessary, interview promising candidates, provide an initial cursory review of biases and conflicts of interest, and submit a slate of primary and alternate nominees for consideration by the secretaries of USDA and HHS. With its experience in the field, USDA and HHS could still be responsible for balancing the final advisory committee and appointing members.

The third party would need to be an organization without a political, economic, or ideological identity. It would need a strong record of hav-

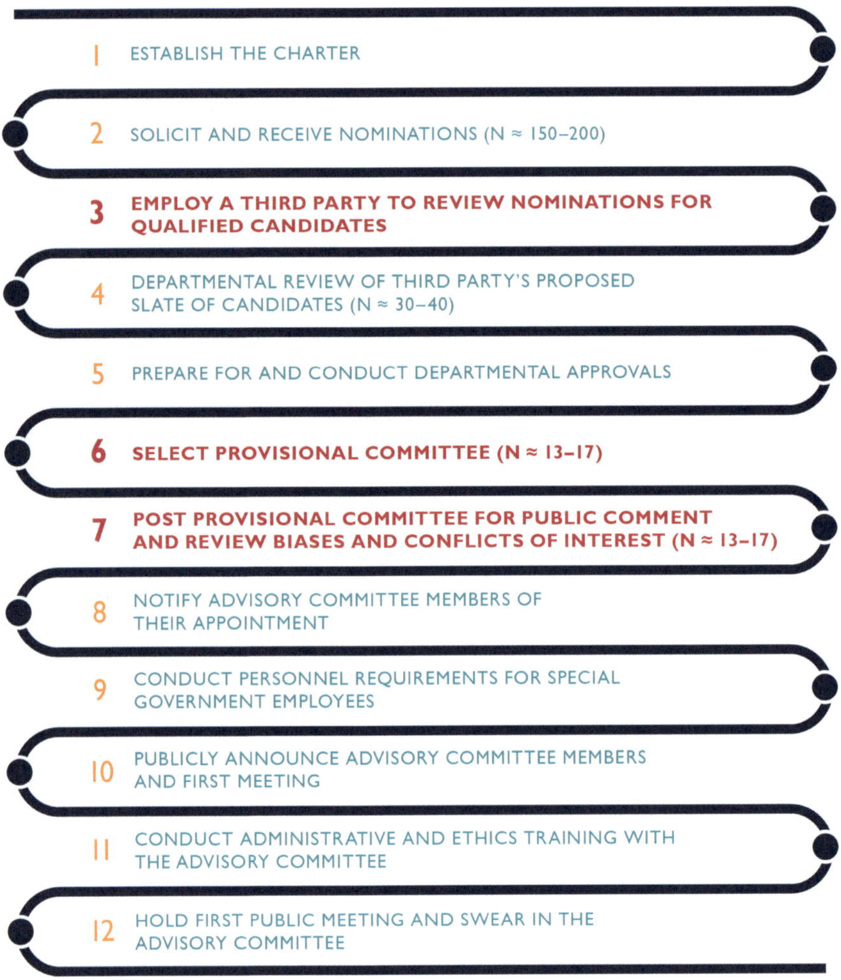
1 ESTABLISH THE CHARTER
2 SOLICIT AND RECEIVE NOMINATIONS (N ≈ 150–200)
3 EMPLOY A THIRD PARTY TO REVIEW NOMINATIONS FOR QUALIFIED CANDIDATES
4 DEPARTMENTAL REVIEW OF THIRD PARTY'S PROPOSED SLATE OF CANDIDATES (N ≈ 30–40)
5 PREPARE FOR AND CONDUCT DEPARTMENTAL APPROVALS
6 SELECT PROVISIONAL COMMITTEE (N ≈ 13–17)
7 POST PROVISIONAL COMMITTEE FOR PUBLIC COMMENT AND REVIEW BIASES AND CONFLICTS OF INTEREST (N ≈ 13–17)
8 NOTIFY ADVISORY COMMITTEE MEMBERS OF THEIR APPOINTMENT
9 CONDUCT PERSONNEL REQUIREMENTS FOR SPECIAL GOVERNMENT EMPLOYEES
10 PUBLICLY ANNOUNCE ADVISORY COMMITTEE MEMBERS AND FIRST MEETING
11 CONDUCT ADMINISTRATIVE AND ETHICS TRAINING WITH THE ADVISORY COMMITTEE
12 HOLD FIRST PUBLIC MEETING AND SWEAR IN THE ADVISORY COMMITTEE

FIGURE S-1 Proposed process for selecting the Dietary Guidelines Advisory Committee.
NOTE: Steps highlighted in red are new, proposed steps.

ing both the theoretical knowledge and practical expertise in the assembly of impartial committees. Since the third party would not be making final selections, it would not necessarily need to be expert in nutrition or dietary guidance, just skilled in evaluating individuals' expertise and experience. It could be a private, nonprofit, or government organization, but should not be part of either sponsoring agency.

This National Academies committee's opinion is that political bias—both the perception and reality—would be reduced by a third party since USDA and HHS would not be involved in narrowing the field of candidates. If the secretaries of USDA and HHS are selecting final nominees from a short list of equally well-qualified, nonconflicted candidates, there is a greater potential that the final DGAC will be neutral. This in fact has the potential to reduce bias but even stronger potential to improve perception. Having the secretaries continue to select the final membership would also remove the need for the external organization to have specific expertise related to the *DGA*, likely resulting in a broader pool of candidates.

There is no absolute guarantee that a third party will reduce bias; there is no evidence to say that a third party would not come up with the same exact committee of experts as assembled by the current process. Additionally, the secretaries of USDA and HHS would remain the appointing authorities. However, to the many critics of the process, a third party would ensure that USDA and HHS were more at an arm's length from the selection of DGAC members. This committee believes that at the very least, this would improve public perception of a more objective process. Another drawback is that this approach would likely have budgetary implications despite some savings in staff time, as well as lengthen the selection process. However, selection of a third party could begin before the charter is filed so as to leave the DGAC with as much time as possible to conduct its work.

Recommendation 1. The secretaries of USDA and HHS should employ an external third party to review and narrow the candidate pool to a list of primary and alternate nominees. Criteria against which nominees are screened should be developed by USDA and HHS for use by the third party.

Membership Criteria and Composition

Critical components in the selection process are the criteria against which they are evaluated and approaches to balancing the advisory committee's overall composition. In the current process, candidates are assessed "based upon their qualifications, level of expertise and knowledge, and ability to contribute to the work to be performed," as well as diversity of "geographic areas, academic institutions, gender, race, ethnicity, and disability." Conflicts of interest and background checks are considered prior to appointment to the advisory committee.

Other factors are likely considered during the balancing process, but they are not explicitly stated. These include willingness to serve; minimal financial and nonfinancial conflicts of interest; biases that can be balanced with those of other members; and prior experience working on advisory committees or panels. Skills need to be reviewed for the group as a whole, as well as individuals. All criteria used in making a final selection ought to be clearly stated. The organization selecting candidates will need to review the collective expertise, experience, and perspectives before making final appointments. Through this deliberative process, the public can be assured that the advisory committee is objective and has the requisite expertise to complete its task.

The composition of the advisory committee ought to be dictated to a great degree by the content areas under review, while also representing a wide variety of perspectives. Ideally, any group of experts with a similar composition could be appointed and derive the same findings. The 2015 DGAC membership balance plan listed but was not limited to a set of 17 specialty areas to be represented. Experts may have experience in one or more of the areas, so a one-to-one match between category of expertise and DGAC members is not required.

In considering the specific areas of expertise needed, the complicated question arose of which should be developed first: the specific questions to be answered by the DGAC or the areas of expertise needed to address the charge? The current process relies on the DGAC to develop priority topics for review rather than for an a priori process to identify which updates and reviews are most critically needed, thus influencing the expertise needed on the DGAC. This National Academies committee discussed the potential value of focusing on specific areas that need revision or updating in the *DGA*. This situation would allow for concentration of expertise in key priority areas rather than comprehensive expertise needed for review of the *complete DGA*. This issue was recognized because of the need to focus on recommendations for pregnant women and children from birth to 24 months in the *2020–2025 DGA*. However, to meet the short timeline for its first report, this National Academies committee was not able to formulate a specific recommendation on this approach or more broadly about the DGAC composition. This issue will be addressed upon a full examination of the DGAC's charge and the overall *DGA* process.

Additional Public Comment Periods

Prior DGACs were criticized primarily for their lack of balance and not necessarily the qualifications of specific individuals. The one formal opportunity for public input during the selection process was in response to a call for nominations.

A reasonable amount of time for feedback is critical to a transparent selection process. The public should have an additional opportunity to comment after the initial solicitation of nominations (see step 7 of Figure S-1). The additional time and resources required for another public comment period was determined to have the significant benefit of increasing transparency during the selection process. Some advisory committees invite the public to comment on all individuals nominated for the activity, while others request comments on a provisional panel before they are officially appointed. Considering the size of the candidate pool (150 to 200 candidates were considered in each of the past three cycles) and the need to focus on the overall composition, an opportunity should be made for the public to provide input on a provisional panel; appointments would be finalized upon consideration of public comments. This would allow the departments to address any concerns raised and encourage transparency.

Recommendation 2. The secretaries of USDA and HHS should make a list of provisional appointees open for public comment—including short biographies and any known conflicts—for a reasonable period of time prior to appointment.

Candid information from the public about proposed members is critical for a deliberative process. However, full transparency in the form of publicly accessible deliberations or posting of public comments about every nominee is not practical given the sensitivity around why someone is or is not considered a strong candidate for DGAC membership. Such a process would likely lead to ad hominem attacks presented in public comments or explanations by USDA or HHS that could result in candidates being maligned in the public press and their reputations damaged, discouraging people from willingly volunteering their time to serve on the DGAC, reducing the pool of qualified candidates.

Biases and Conflicts of Interest

Biases and conflicts of interest may unduly influence the deliberations and outcomes of an advisory committee. The perception of biases and conflicts of interest can also undermine the public's trust in the process. It is therefore critical that these biases and influences be discussed prior to appointment. But given the breadth of this National Academies committee's definitions of biases and conflicts of interest to include nonfinancial conflicts, the committee does not believe these influences can be eliminated *entirely*. As such, those who have had relationships with industry or issue-specific advocates in the recent past could participate fairly on a panel if the nature of the relationship was incidental to the work of the panel. However, strict policies must be made publicly available explaining how such conflicts will be identified and managed.

To identify conflicts, the federal Office of Government Ethics Form 450, which is currently used for the DGAC, was found to cover financial conflicts of interest adequately. However, since the Office of Government Ethics only reviews financial conflicts, no explicit, formal steps were identified for candidates to disclose nonfinancial conflicts or biases. To enhance transparency, a form should be developed and used for the disclosure of relevant nonfinancial conflicts of interest and biases. Ethics officers not involved in the development of the *DGA* should independently judge the presence of conflicts. A detailed description of how biases and conflicts of interest would be identified should be made publicly available as part of a policy concerning bias and conflict of interest.

Potential biases and conflicts of interest ought to be disclosed at varying levels to three audiences: the appropriate ethics officers; other members of the specific activity, in this case, DGAC members; and to the public to the extent possible. Any potential biases or conflicts should be shared with ethics officers. Disclosure should also be made revealing sources of conflicts to all other DGAC members so they can better understand the basis for each other's positions. Finally, an abstraction of conflicts of interest deemed to be significant ought to be shared with the public, including sources of funding, consultancies, and other relationships as appropriate.

Management of biases and conflicts of interest are as important as their identification. Many tools exist to manage conflicts of interest. For example, exemptions could be made in instances where the potential conflict is deemed too remote or inconsequential to significantly influence an individual's judgment, or waivers could be granted that would allow for varying ranges of participation. Changes to the advisory committee's structure could also be adopted to minimize the effect of any undue influence during its work. Individuals could also choose to resign from a disqualifying activity or divest property. These and other approaches are often used to mitigate the effect of activities deemed to be actual or perceived conflicts. A certification describing management plans put in place should be issued with the advisory committee's final report.

Recommendation 3. The secretaries of USDA and HHS should disclose how provisional nominees' biases and conflicts of interest are identified and managed by

- **a. Creating and publicly posting a policy and form to explicitly disclose financial and nonfinancial biases and conflicts;**
- **b. Developing a management plan for addressing biases and conflicts for the panel as a whole and individuals, as needed;**

c. **Certifying that a federal ethics officer independently reviewed and judged the advisory committee's biases and conflicts of interest; and by**
d. **Documenting how conflicts of interest were managed in the Dietary Guidelines Advisory Committee report.**

A CONTINUOUSLY LEARNING SELECTION PROCESS

USDA and HHS will need to dynamically improve the DGAC selection process to drive toward positive change and contribute to enhanced trustworthiness of the *DGA*. Sustained, optimal performance of a process is the product of systematic quality improvement activities. Development of systemic quality improvement will allow future DGAC selection processes to be grounded in evidence. However, development of a true system for quality improvement takes time and commitment. This National Academies committee recognizes that both development of a system for quality improvement and changes to the DGAC selection process will not be immediate. Actions could be taken in the short term and are suggested at three levels: the selection process as a whole, the structure of the advisory committee, and advisory committee functions. Improvements should be made as evidence about the selection process evolves and becomes available. A full discussion of a continuously learning process will be presented in this National Academies committee's second report.

Recommendation 4. The secretaries of USDA and HHS should adopt a system for continuous process improvement to enhance outcomes and performance of the Dietary Guidelines Advisory Committee selection process.

1

Introduction

Every system is perfectly designed to get the results it gets.

—Paul Batalden

Federal advice to the public on nutrition and diet is intended to reflect the state of the science and deliver the most reliable recommendations according to the best available evidence. This advice, presented in the *Dietary Guidelines for Americans* (*DGA*), underpins all federal nutrition policies and programs and is updated every 5 years. The process to create the guidelines is not a simple one, and it changes as the science evolves. Much has been accomplished to improve how the science is evaluated and translated into the *DGA*, such as the establishment of the Nutrition Evidence Library to conduct evidence-based reviews. The target population for the *DGA* will also expand in the 2020–2025 edition to include recommendations for all Americans by including pregnant women and children from birth to 2 years.

Despite the many accomplishments, recent challenges to federal nutrition guidance prompted Congress to question the process by which food and nutrition guidance is developed (Conaway, 2015; Hartzler et al., 2015). To address these complicated questions, Congress mandated a review of the entire process used to develop the *DGA*.[1]

[1]Consolidated Appropriations Act, 2016, Public Law 114-113, 114th Cong. (December 18, 2015), 129 Stat. 2280–2281.

THE *DIETARY GUIDELINES FOR AMERICANS*

The *DGA* is a report that provides nutritional and dietary information to promote health and prevent disease (HHS/USDA, 2015). To help Americans make healthy food choices, the U.S. Department of Agriculture (USDA) and the U.S. Department of Health and Human Services (HHS) jointly review and update the guidelines every 5 years to reflect "the preponderance of the scientific and medical knowledge which is current at the time the report is prepared."[2] Since the first edition in 1980, the guidelines have served as the basis for all federal nutrition policies and nutrition assistance programs, as well as nutrition education programs (see Box 1-1). The process to develop the guidelines has evolved over time in an effort to develop gold standard guidelines.

The guidelines are developed through a multistep process developed by USDA and HHS. USDA and HHS receive input from a scientific advisory committee, other federal agencies, and the public (see Figure 1-1).

First, a charter is filed with Congress to establish a scientific advisory committee, known as the Dietary Guidelines Advisory Committee (DGAC). The advisory committee comprises nationally recognized experts responsible for independently evaluating the scientific evidence to inform revisions to the current policy or suggest new guidance. Its conclusions are submitted to the secretaries of USDA and HHS as the *Scientific Report of the Dietary Guidelines Advisory Committee*. The DGAC's report serves as the scientific basis for the *DGA*, but its conclusions are advisory in nature only; the scientific report does not constitute draft policy.

The secretaries then solicit comments on the DGAC report from the public and other federal agencies. Next, the *DGA* writing team—made up of staff from USDA and HHS—collects, assesses, and reviews these comments as it develops the next edition of the *DGA*. The draft undergoes a series of internal departmental reviews, including reviews by more than 100 subject-matter experts from the federal government, and revisions prior to approval by the secretaries. Finally, the *DGA* is published publicly with the primary audience being policymakers and health professionals who then implement the guidelines through programs supported by federal, state, and local governments.

When the *Scientific Report of the 2015 Dietary Guidelines Advisory Committee* was released in February 2015, more than 29,000 written public comments were submitted. Only five of these public comments focused

---

[2]National Nutrition Monitoring and Related Research Act of 1990, Public Law 101-445, 101st Cong. (October 22, 1990) 7 U.S.C. 5341, 104 Stat. 1042–1044. The departments are required to act within the National Nutrition Monitoring and Related Research Act of 1990, Agricultural Act of 2014, Federal Advisory Committee Act of 1972, and the Consolidated Appropriations Act of 2001 ("Data Quality Act") (USDA/HHS, 2016a).

on the membership of the DGAC, stating that future DGACs should include food scientists, more registered dietitians, and other health professionals and practitioners (HHS, 2016). Critiques of the report itself and the process used—both in support of and against the conclusions—were raised for a wide range of topics. Comments questioning the report focused largely on the DGAC's scope with some suggesting that it was too broad. Also questioned were aspects of the *process* it used to evaluate the scientific evidence. The DGAC was criticized for not having had the charge or expertise to make some of its recommendations, such as those related to sustainable diets and tax policy (Hartzler et al., 2015; Jack, 2016; Kovich, 2016; Merrigan et al., 2015). Questions were also raised regarding the evidence used and the comprehensiveness of the literature reviewed (Dabrowska, 2016; Heimowitz, 2016; Hentges, 2016; Mozzaffarian, 2016; Teicholz, 2015). Following an examination of these public comments, the House Committee on Agriculture held a hearing where the secretaries of USDA and HHS were asked to clarify, among other things, that the DGAC report was based in science and that sustainability concerns were outside the scope of the DGAC. Controversy arose again in January 2016 when the *Dietary Guidelines for Americans 2015–2020, Eighth Edition,* was released. Those critical of the document focused, among other things, on the process by which the DGAC's scientific report was translated into the policy document (the *DGA*) (Walsh, 2016; Willett, 2016).

Other comments were made on February 19, 2016, when USDA invited 40 stakeholders to voice support or concern for the process for developing the *DGA*. Ten professional organizations were represented, as well as 18 members of the food industry, and 12 individuals with various background and professional associations. Specific to the membership issue of the DGAC, conflict of interest was raised as a prime area of concern among stakeholders who commented on the selection process, with views ranging from no potential members having any ties to the food industry at all, to acceptance of past conflicts of interest. There was general agreement among commenters that the composition of the DGAC should be diversified and expanded to include additional expertise including government, food industry, academia, nongovernmental organizations, and consumer representatives.[3] It was noted that no single sector should have undue influence on the selection process. Some stakeholders supported the current selection process, and others offered suggestions such as publicizing selection criteria and any relevant conflicts of interest, as well as using public nominations for selecting the advisory committee (USDA, 2016b).

[3]Specific areas of expertise called for, mentioned by more than three stakeholders, included pregnancy and birth to 24 months, registered dietitians, food industry, consumer behavior, food systems, food technology, nutrition, pediatrics.

BOX 1-1
Applications of the *Dietary Guidelines for Americans*

The key recommendations provided in the *Dietary Guidelines for Americans* (*DGA*) are intended to be translated into action to help Americans consume healthful diets. One of the main functions of the guidelines is to provide food-based guidance for federal nutrition programs. These include but are not limited to the National School Lunch Program; the School Breakfast Program; the Special Supplemental Nutrition Program for Women, Infants, and Children (WIC); and the Child and Adult Care Food Program (CACFP). Applications of the *DGA*, however, include policies, programs, and outreach material at the federal, state, and local levels. Three specific examples are described below.

Aligning School Meal Standards with the *DGA*

As two nutrition programs administered by USDA, the National School Lunch Program and the School Breakfast Program must provide meals that are aligned with the *DGA*. The federal standards used for meal planning for these programs are assessed for adherence to the latest edition of the guidelines and, if needed, adjusted accordingly. The release of the *2010 DGA*, for example, led to establishing vegetables as their own component, separate from fruits, in the National School Lunch Program. The Final Rule further specified that all vegetable subgroups defined in the *2010 DGA* (dark green, red/orange, beans and peas [legumes], starchy, and other) must be provided over the course of a week.[a] Another change included the National School Lunch Program and School Breakfast Program after the release of the *2010 DGA* was that only grains qualifying as "whole grain-rich" may be served.

Not all updates to the *DGA* key recommendations lead to substantial programmatic changes, and consideration is given to the feasibility of implementation. USDA determined that the standards for the National School Lunch Program and School Breakfast Program based on the *2010 DGA* were consistent with the *2015–2020 DGA*.[b] The Final Rule noted, however, that compliance with the *2015–2020 DGA* recommendation of limiting added sugar to no more than 10 percent of calories was not readily implementable with respect to competitive foods sold in the school setting. To put this recommendation into operation, the contribution of added sugars to total calories of each product would have to be known. This information is not currently listed on Nutrition Facts labels and is challenging to discern at present. Until added sugars are separately listed on Nutrition Facts labels (see next page), the standard for sugars will remain based on its contribution to the food products' total weight.

Updating the Nutrition Facts Label

In May 2016, the U.S. Food and Drug Administration (FDA) announced changes to the Nutrition Facts labels intended to reflect current scientific evidence and help consumers make informed choices.[c] One revision is to list the amount of total sugars that come from added sugars. FDA cites the revision as providing alignment with the *2015–2020 DGA*'s key recommendation regarding added sugars (FDA, 2016).

Another revision affects the percent daily values. The percent daily values show how much a serving of the food contributes to reference intake levels for a nutrient. FDA updated the daily reference value for sodium, guided in part by the *2010 DGA*; the key recommendation for sodium did not change with the latest version of the *DGA*. The revisions to the Nutrition Facts labels are scheduled to be fully implemented by all manufacturers by July 2019.

Establishing Policies at the State Level

Although its primary role is to guide federal nutrition-related efforts, the *DGA* is also used by policy makers and health professionals throughout the country. In 2009, Massachusetts became the first state to enact a statewide food procurement policy for state agencies.[d] The resulting nutrition standards developed by the Massachusetts Department of Health were based on the *DGA, 2005* (Massachusetts Executive Office of Health and Human Services, 2016), and have been reevaluated to ensure alignment with subsequent editions (Massachusetts Department of Public Health, 2012). Standards were set for each food group (e.g., milks provided to individuals 2 years and older must be low-fat or nonfat) and food preparation (e.g., elimination of deep fryers). Similarly, state agencies in Washington were required to begin implementing healthy food service guidelines as of July 1, 2014.[e] From this executive order came the *Healthy Nutrition Guidelines* (Washington State Department of Health, 2014), which follow the *2010 DGA*, and are provided for vending, meetings and events, cafeterias, and institutions.

---

[a]7 C.F.R. § 210 and 220, 2012.

[b]7 C.F.R. § 210 and 220, 2016.

[c]21 C.F.R. § 101, 2016.

[d]Massachusetts Executive Order 509, Establishing Nutrition Standards for Food Purchased and Served by State Agencies (2009).

[e]Washington Executive Order 13-06, Improving the Health and Productivity of State Employees and Access to Healthy Foods in State Facilities (2013).

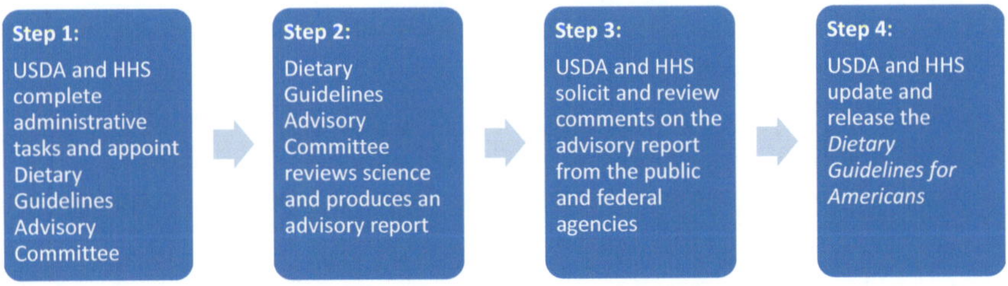

FIGURE 1-1 Primary steps for updating the *Dietary Guidelines for Americans.*
SOURCE: Abstracted from USDA, 2016a.

EVALUATION BY THE NATIONAL ACADEMIES OF SCIENCES, ENGINEERING, AND MEDICINE

In response to concerns raised about the process to produce the *2015–2020 DGA*, Congress directed USDA to engage with the National Academies of Sciences, Engineering, and Medicine (the National Academies) to appoint a committee to conduct a comprehensive evaluation of the *processes* used to establish the *DGA* (see Box 1-2 for the statement of task). Importantly, the committee is not evaluating the substance of the guidelines or their use; its charge is to *assess the process*. The questions in the statement of task are to be divided and addressed in two reports.

This current report responds to the first part of the task: "How the advisory committee selection process can be improved to provide more transparency, eliminate bias, and include committee members with a range of viewpoints," for the purpose of informing the 2020 cycle, which is scheduled to begin in early 2017. The phrase "eliminate bias" is interpreted to mean "minimize bias," as complete elimination of bias may not be possible; this reframing of the charge was accepted by USDA (USDA/HHS, 2016b).

The findings and conclusions contained herein respond only to the first question in the statement of task; remaining questions will be answered in a second report. Although most of the evidence and analysis related to the other questions will be reserved for the second report, some issues related to the second report had to be included in the present report when needed to address the advisory committee selection process. For example, the Agricultural Act of 2014 requested that the *DGA* expand to include people across the life span, adding guidance for pregnant women and children from birth to 24 months. Although this expansion is included in the statement of task under parts 2–4, not part 1, this significant change to the *DGA*—and by extension to the DGAC—may affect the composition

BOX 1-2
Statement of Task

An ad hoc committee will undertake an 18-month study to review the entire process used to establish the Advisory Committee for the Dietary Guidelines for Americans (DGAC) and the subsequent development of the *DGA*, most recently revised pursuant to section 301 of the National Nutrition Monitoring and Related Research Act of 1990 (7 U.S.C. § 5341). The committee will review the current processes for each of the following:

1. How the advisory committee selection process can be improved to provide more transparency, eliminate bias, and include committee members with a range of viewpoints;
2. How the Nutrition Evidence Library (NEL) is compiled and utilized, including whether NEL reviews and other systematic reviews and data analysis are conducted according to rigorous and objective scientific standards;
3. How systematic reviews are conducted on long-standing *DGA* recommendations, including whether scientific studies are included from scientists with a range of viewpoints; and
4. How the *DGA* can better prevent chronic disease, ensure nutritional sufficiency for all Americans, and accommodate a range of individual factors, including age, gender, and metabolic health.

The committee will produce a short report that includes a review of question 1 and, as needed, recommendations based on existing best practices for selecting a scientific advisory committee to inform development of the *DGA*. A final report will be produced that includes the committee's review of questions 2–4 and, as needed, recommendations based on existing practices for

- Conducting and/or including rigorous and objective nutrition systematic reviews and other data analyses to support the development of the *DGA*;
- Supporting an expanded life-span approach, specifically dietary guidance for infants up to 24 months and pregnant women (per the Agricultural Act of 2014);
- Effectively applying the *DGA* to prevent diet-related chronic disease in the United States using existing implementation and evaluation frameworks; and
- Identifying the role of the *DGA* in coordinating with and supporting nutrition guidance for disease treatment (that may also address age, gender, metabolic health, and nutritional sufficiency) developed by other federal agencies.

The committee's recommendations will conform to the specifications of the National Nutrition Monitoring and Related Research Act, Federal Advisory Committee Act, Data Quality Act, and align with the current infrastructure, availability of resources, and collaborative relationships led by the USDA Center for Nutrition Policy and Promotion (study sponsor) and the HHS Office of Disease Prevention and Health Promotion. The committee will not conduct systematic reviews of nutrition science, nor evaluate the content or scientific justification of current or previous editions of the *DGA*.

or structure of the DGAC. As part of an overall, comprehensive review of the process to update the *DGA*, additional findings and recommendations about the selection process may be made as part of this committee's second report. Additionally, some of the questions relevant to the selection process, such as how specific priority areas are determined and how the DGAC's conclusions are considered in the final *DGA*, will be explored in this committee's second report.

Committee Methods

The National Academies appointed 14 members to the Committee to Review the Process to Update the *Dietary Guidelines for Americans* to respond to a congressional request.[4] To assess the advisory committee selection process, this National Academies committee met in person once and convened in closed session three times. Its discussions also benefited from engaging with the public by holding two open information-gathering sessions (see Appendix B). One public comment session was held, where members of the public were invited to address the committee; those who did make a statement included representatives of industry, professional organizations, and advocacy groups. Additionally, the committee solicited input from the public about what they believed to be the most important change that could be made to the selection process. Statements and comments were received by this National Academies committee from a variety of perspectives (see Appendix B). All statements were considered over the course of the committee's deliberations.

Chapter 2 of this report reviews the current process for establishing and operating the DGAC, which is required to act within the Federal Advisory Committee Act. The chapter describes the relevant provisions of the act, and how they affect the establishment of the charter, bylaws, and operating procedures.

The committee sought to ground its work in as much evidence as possible. An evaluation was conducted of the processes for convening other advisory committees. The goal of this search was to identify promising practices and to learn from the wide variation of processes used. A full discussion of this search is presented in Chapter 3.

This National Academies committee also reviewed the published literature to explore the role of conflicts of interest in the development of advisory committees and guidelines (see Appendix A for literature search methods). The ultimate goal of limiting and managing conflicts of interest is to develop a trustworthy process and create reliable guidelines. Ideally,

---

[4]Consolidated Appropriations Act, 2016, Public Law 114-113, 114th Cong. (December 18, 2015), 129 Stat. 2280–2281.

the guidelines, which have been developed with minimal bias, will be trustworthy, leading people to follow the recommendations put forth, which subsequently would lead to improved health outcomes. Management strategies are discussed in more detail in Chapter 4, as well as other opportunities to build trust with the public.

Finally, Chapter 5 discusses the need to continuously update the selection process as new evidence becomes available.

REFERENCES

Conaway, M. 2015. The science in our diet. *U.S. News & World Report.* http://www.usnews.com/opinion/articles/2015/10/05/why-the-science-behind-the-dietary-guidelines-matters (accessed October 3, 2017).

Dabrowska, A. 2016. Dietary Guidelines for Americans: *Frequently asked questions.* R44360. Washington, DC: Congressional Research Service.

FDA (U.S. Food and Drug Administration). 2016. *Changes to the Nutrition Facts label.* http://www.fda.gov/Food/GuidanceRegulation/GuidanceDocumentsRegulatoryInformation/LabelingNutrition/ucm385663.htm (accessed October 3, 2017).

Hartzler, V., M. Conaway, J. Walorski, K. Noem, and D. Webster. 2015. *Letter from Members of Congress to the Honorable Tom Vilsack, Secretary of Agriculture and the Honorable Sylvia Mathews Burwell, Secretary of Health and Human Services (March 31, 2015).* http://agriculture.house.gov/uploadedfiles/ag_dietaryguidelineslettertosecsvilsackburwell.pdf (accessed October 3, 2017).

Heimowitz, C. 2016 (unpublished). *Comments presented at USDA* Dietary Guidelines for Americans *listening sessions: Atkins Nutritionals.* Washington, DC, February 19, 2016.

Hentges, E. 2016 (unpublished). *Comments presented at USDA* Dietary Guidelines for Americans *listening sessions: International Life Sciences Institute.* Washington, DC, February 19, 2016.

HHS (U.S. Department of Health and Human Services). 2016. Public comments on the scientific report of the 2015 Dietary Guidelines Advisory Committee. https://health.gov/dietaryguidelines/dga2015/comments/advisory-report-summary.asp (accessed October 4, 2017).

HHS/USDA (U.S. Department of Health and Human Services/U.S. Department of Agriculture). 2015. Dietary Guidelines for Americans *2015–2020: Eighth edition.* https://health.gov/dietaryguidelines/2015/guidelines (accessed October 4, 2017).

Jack, M. 2016 (unpublished). *Comments presented at USDA* Dietary Guidelines for Americans *listening sessions: American Beverage Association.* Washington, DC, February 19, 2016.

Kovich, D. 2016 (unpublished). *Comments presented at USDA* Dietary Guidelines for Americans *listening sessions: National Pork Producers Council.* Washington, DC, February 19, 2016.

Massachusetts Department of Public Health. 2012. *Massachusetts State Agency Food Standards: Requirements and recommendations.* http://www.mass.gov/eohhs/docs/dph/mass-in-motion/eo509-state-agency-food-standards.pdf (accessed October 4, 2017).

Massachusetts Executive Office of Health and Human Services. 2016. *Tools and resources for implementation of Executive Order 509.* http://www.mass.gov/eohhs/gov/departments/dph/programs/community-health/mass-in-motion/about-mim/components/tools-and-resources-for-executive-order-509.html (accessed October 4, 2017).

Merrigan, K., T. Griffin, P. Wilde, K. Robien, J. Goldberg, and W. Dietz. 2015. Designing a sustainable diet. *Science* 350(6257):165-166.

Mozzaffarian, D. 2016 (unpublished). *Comments presented at USDA* Dietary Guidelines for Americans *listening sessions.* Washington, DC, February 19, 2016.

Teicholz, N. 2015. The scientific report guiding the US dietary guidelines: Is it scientific? *British Medical Journal* 351:h4962.

USDA (U.S. Department of Agriculture). 2016a (unpublished). *Understanding the committee's charge: A discussion with the sponsor.* Presentation to the Committee to Review the Process to Update the *Dietary Guidelines for Americans.*

USDA. 2016b. *Dietary Guidelines for Americans* Listening Sessions: Transcript. https://www.cnpp.usda.gov/sites/default/files/dietary_guidelines_for_americans/ListeningSessionTranscript-2-19-16.pdf (accessed October 4, 2017).

USDA/HHS (U.S. Department of Agriculture/U.S. Department of Health and Human Services). 2016a (unpublished). Dietary Guidelines for Americans: *Process brief, sections 1–3.* Prepared for the Committee to Review the Process to Update the *Dietary Guidelines for Americans.*

USDA/HHS. 2016b (unpublished). *HMD follow-up questions for USDA.* Response to Committee to Review the Process to Update the *Dietary Guidelines for Americans.*

Walsh, D. 2016 (unpublished). *Comments presented at USDA* Dietary Guidelines for Americans *listening sessions: Snack Food Association.* Washington, DC, February 19, 2016.

Washington State Department of Health. 2014. *Healthy nutrition guidelines: Implementation guide for agencies, sites and vendors.* Healthy Communities. (DOH 340-224).

Willett, W. 2016 (unpublished). *Comments presented at USDA* Dietary Guidelines for Americans *listening sessions.* Washington, DC, February 19, 2016.

2

The Dietary Guidelines Advisory Committee Process

A BRIEF HISTORY

In 1977, the U.S. Senate Select Committee on Nutrition and Human Needs recommended a set of dietary goals for Americans, calling for the public to expend as much or more energy (kcals) as it consumes, and suggesting nutrient- and food-based targets. When those goals were publicly released, industry and the scientific community questioned whether the recommendations could be supported by available science. To provide the public with authoritative guidance on diet and health, the U.S. Department of Agriculture (USDA) and the U.S. Department of Health and Human Services (HHS) (then called the U.S. Department of Health, Education, and Welfare) convened scientists from within the departments and released a set of principles in the 1980 report *Nutrition and Your Health: Dietary Guidelines for Americans*, the first edition of the dietary guidelines. Like the 1977 report, the 1980 report suggested a causal relationship between the guidelines and health that also sparked questions about whether sufficient science was available to make these recommendations. To address those concerns, a 1983 congressional report directed that a scientific advisory committee of external experts be convened to review the evidence and suggest updates to the 1980 report. Those recommended revisions informed the development of the second edition of the *Dietary Guidelines for Americans* (*DGA*; 1985). Congress indicated that advisory committees should continue to be reestablished to review relevant scientific data and make recommendations on appropriate changes to the secretaries of USDA and HHS.[1] As a result, an advisory committee has been an explicit part of the Dietary Guidelines process for more than 30 years, more commonly known as the Dietary Guidelines Advisory Committee (DGAC) (HHS/USDA, 2013).

The role of diet in preventing chronic disease was questioned after conflicting reports were released on the effectiveness of dietary recommendations on the public's health. These reports made clear that a universal standard of scientific evidence regarding nutrition is needed (GAO, 1984). Three landmark publications—*The Surgeon General's Report on Nutrition and Health* (HHS, 1988), *Diet and Health: Implications for Reducing Chronic Disease Risk* (NRC, 1989), and *How Should the Recommended Dietary Allowances Be Revised?* (IOM, 1994)—set the stage for a public conversation about the role of diet in reducing risk of chronic disease, food components related to health benefits, and evaluation of risk from both nutritional deficiency and excess as contemporary public health concerns. As an outcome, federal nutrition policy began to evolve, incorporating the concept of the whole diet and the role of food-based dietary patterns into guidance for the public about diet and health.

ESTABLISHMENT OF A FEDERAL ADVISORY COMMITTEE

The DGAC is established pursuant to the National Nutrition Monitoring Act and governed by the Federal Advisory Committee Act (FACA), which directs the establishment, operation, oversight, and termination of advisory committees to the executive branch of the federal government.[2] One key goal of the act is to ensure advice is objective and accessible to the public.[3] The act is generally not prescriptive, but rather it provides executive branch agencies and/or departments (hereafter referred to as agencies when referencing FACA) with the flexibility to develop their own processes. Agencies have discretion over the particular processes they put in place where the act is silent. Agencies are also required to develop administrative guidelines that describe how they will implement FACA at their agency; while the content of these guidelines is at the agency's discretion, they must be consistent with FACA. To comply with FACA, a number of administrative processes must be followed to establish the DGAC, which is installed at the discretion of the secretaries of USDA and HHS, including filing of a charter and developing a plan to fairly balance membership (see Box 2-1).

---

[1]U.S. House of Representatives Conference Committee. 100th Cong., 1st sess., H. Rep. 498, 1987.

[2]Federal Advisory Committee Act, 1972, Public Law 92-463. 92nd Cong., 86 Stat. 770.

[3]Advice must come from groups that include at least one nonfederal member.

BOX 2-1
Federal Advisory Committee Establishment

Federal advisory committees can be categorized into two broad groups: discretionary and nondiscretionary. As defined in 41 C.F.R. § 102-3.25:

- *Discretionary advisory committees* are "established under the authority of an agency head or authorized by statute. An advisory committee referenced in general (nonspecific) authorizing language or congressional committee report language is discretionary, and its establishment or termination is within the legal discretion of an agency head."
- *Nondiscretionary advisory committees* are "either required by statute or by presidential directive. A nondiscretionary advisory committee required by statute generally is identified specifically in a statute by name, purpose, or functions, and its establishment or termination is beyond the legal discretion of an agency head."

Regardless of establishment authority, all federal advisory committees must comply with the Federal Advisory Committee Act and the 2001 Final Rule on federal advisory committee management. The operational requirements for discretionary and nondiscretionary committees are the same, unless otherwise specified in statute.

In establishing, renewing, or reestablishing a discretionary federal advisory committee, agencies are required to

- *Consult with the committee management secretariat.* During the consultation, the agency must justify why the committee is needed, explain how the function of the committee is nonduplicative, and describe how the membership of the committee will be fairly balanced.
- *Publish a notice in the* Federal Register. The agency must publish a notice in the *Federal Register* for federal advisory committees being established or reestablished at least 15 days before the committee's charter is filed, except for instances when the committee management secretariat has approved a shorter duration. Committees that are being renewed also have to publish a notice in the *Federal Register*, but it can occur concurrently with the filing of the charter.
- *File a charter with the appropriate authorities.* Charters must be filed with the agency head, Senate and House of Representatives standing committees with legislative jurisdiction over the agency, the Library of Congress, and the committee management secretariat.

Nondiscretionary committees, in contrast, are not required to consult with the committee management secretariat; however, a consultation is strongly encouraged for both the charter and the plan for how membership balance will be achieved. Nondiscretionary committees are, however, required to file a charter with the same authorities noted above for discretionary committees. Unless otherwise specified in legislation, all charters expire 2 years after their effective date and must be renewed if the committee's duration is longer than 2 years.

BOX 2-2
Categories of Federal Advisory Committees: Members and Related Ethical Considerations

A member of a federal advisory committee falls under one of the following categories: special government employee, regular government employee, representative, or ex officio. This designation depends on whether the member is providing expertise as either a government employee or temporary government employee, or is providing the perspective of a group. Members can also be part of a federal advisory committee by virtue of the position they hold either within or outside of the government.

Special government employee: An officer or employee who is retained, designated, appointed, or employed to perform temporary duties for the executive or legislative branch of the U.S. government, with or without compensation, for not more than 130 days during any period of 365 consecutive days.[a] Individuals who serve on advisory committees as special government employees are appointed to a federal advisory committee to exercise their own individual best judgment on behalf of the federal government. It is expected that special government employees will discuss and deliberate in a manner that is free from conflicts of interest.

Regular government employee: An individual who is an employee or officer of the federal government.

Representative: An individual who is not a federal employee, who is selected for membership on a federal advisory committee for the purpose of obtaining the point of view or perspective of nongovernmental entities or of a recognizable

Federal advisory committees can be composed of members from one or more of the following categories: special government employees, regular government employees, representative members, and ex officio members (see descriptions in Box 2-2).

While USDA and HHS develop the guidelines jointly, the administrative lead for a particular edition of the guidelines is responsible for following the appropriate processes (e.g., USDA is the lead for the 2020–2025 report). A memorandum of understanding is put in place between the two departments to provide a framework for this collaborative relationship. The following sections describe the relevant FACA processes and HHS and USDA's interpretation of the law in the development of the 2015–2020 edition of the *DGA*. The process includes filing the charter and submitting the membership balance plan. Other administrative tasks USDA and HHS complete include updating bylaws, updating the charge, and preparing a database for public comments (USDA/HHS, 2016a).

group of persons (e.g., industry sector, labor unions, or environmental groups). It is expected that representatives will represent a particular bias.

Ex officio: An individual who is selected to serve on the federal advisory committee strictly by virtue of holding a specific governmental or organizational office, title, or other specified position.

Members designated as regular or special government employees are subject to federal laws regarding conflicts of interest and ethical standards. Regular and special government employees are required to complete financial disclosures, which are used by the agency to assess the potential for a financial conflict of interest. Special government employees may be granted a waiver if the appointing authority determines and certifies that the need for the individual's service on the advisory committee outweighs the potential for conflicts created by the financial interest.[b] Federal advisory committee members who are selected to represent a viewpoint of a specific group, in contrast, are known to have biases. Such members are not government employees and thus are not subject to the criminal laws regarding financial conflicts of interest.

Members who are not federal government employees or officers may be eligible for compensation for serving on the federal advisory committee. The appointing authority determines whether advisory committee members are paid, and if so, at what level according to the government general schedule pay scale.

[a] 18 U.S.C. § 202.
[b] 18 U.S.C. § 208(b)(3).
SOURCES: GSA, 2016; OGE, 2016.

Charter

To establish a federal advisory committee to advise an agency or federal official in the executive branch of government, FACA requires a charter be filed with the agency head; standing committees of the Senate and House having legislative jurisdiction of the agency; the Library of Congress; and the committee management secretariat. The charter outlines the mission and scope for advisory committees and includes the following: (1) Committee's official designation; (2) Authority; (3) Objectives and scope of activities; (4) Description of duties; (5) Agency or official to whom the committee reports; (6) Support; (7) Estimated annual operating costs and staff years; (8) Designated federal officer; (9) Estimated number and frequency of meetings; (10) Duration; (11) Termination; (12) Membership and designation; (13) Subcommittees; (14) Recordkeeping; and (15) Filing date (GSA, 2011b).[4]

The DGAC is a discretionary committee, which means that it is established by either the secretary of USDA and HHS; the agency with administrative lead switches with every edition of the *DGA*. The decision to establish or terminate the DGAC lies with the respective secretary. The main objective listed in the charter of the 2015 DGAC was "to provide independent, science-based advice and recommendations for development of the *Dietary Guidelines for Americans, 2015*" (Secretary of Health and Human Services, 2013). The committee's report is described as the basis for the policy document, although the committee's work is advisory only. The charter instructs the committee to take new scientific evidence and current resource documents into consideration of its scientific recommendations. Notably, the DGAC is directed to state its rationale in the presentation of its conclusions.

As part of the process, USDA and HHS each appoint co-executive secretaries from their respective agencies to support the work of the advisory committee and ensure it stays within its charge. For the 2015 advisory committee, a total of four co-executive secretaries, two from USDA and two from HHS, were appointed.[5] One of the officials from the lead agency serves as the designated federal officer to oversee management and support services and submit FACA reporting requirements.

The "membership and designation" field states not only the expected number of committee members but also the categories of expertise to be represented. The 2015 advisory committee was proposed to consist of 13 to 17 members, led by a chair, and potential for a vice chair and/or cochairs. In the end, 15 members were appointed by the secretaries of HHS and USDA, led by a chair and vice chair. One member stepped down from the committee after 3 months and was not replaced, leaving a total of 14 members. Members were appointed for the duration of the project. All members of the 2015 DGAC were classified as special government employees (see Box 2-2), meaning that all members were chosen to represent themselves and use their own judgment on behalf of the federal government, and were not representing a group or entity. In accordance with FACA, the advisory committee is limited to 2 years to complete its work.

---

[4]The authority, designated federal officer, membership and designation, subcommittees, and recordkeeping sections "are not explicitly required (at this time) but improve the overall charter and provide valuable additional information for interested parties" (GSA, 2011b).

[5]The USDA undersecretaries of food, nutrition, and consumer services and research, education, and economics appoint one representative from the Center for Nutrition Policy and Promotion and one from the Agricultural Research Service. The two representatives from the Health and Human Services Office of Disease Prevention and Health Promotion are appointed by the assistant secretary for health.

Expertise sought for the 2015 DGAC as listed in the charter included but was not limited to cardiovascular disease; type 2 diabetes; overweight and obesity; osteoporosis; cancer; pediatrics; gerontology; maternal/gestational nutrition; epidemiology; general medicine; energy balance, which includes physical activity; nutrient bioavailability; nutrition biochemistry and physiology; food processing science, safety, and technology; public health; nutrition education and behavior change; and/or nutrition-related systematic review methodology (Secretary of Health and Human Services, 2013). These categories of expertise are developed by the departments and are revised with each charter.

Advisory committee members do not receive payment for their service with the exception of per diem and reimbursed travel expenses. Estimated annual operating costs to support the 2015 advisory committee were $400,000. A total of 4.4 full-time equivalents were projected to support the DGAC. Additional costs borne by the departments for administrative support and staff time were not included in these estimates (USDA/HHS, 2016a).

The charter clearly provides the advisory committee's authority to establish subcommittees and working groups. These groups may only provide recommendations to the parent committee and may not report directly to a federal official. The 2015 advisory committee split itself into three initial working groups. Upon developing its direction, the DGAC broke into five topic-specific subcommittees and four working/writing groups.[6] Under the 2015 charter, the DGAC was authorized to identify and use nonmember consultants who did not vote on the final report. Two subcommittees of the 2015 DGAC engaged with three consultants who were expert in the respective subcommittees' work. Consultants were trained and cleared through a formal federal process similar to the one the DGAC members underwent (HHS/USDA, 2015, part C).

Membership Balance Plan

As part of its compliance with FACA, agencies must ensure the membership of a federal advisory committee is "fairly balanced in terms of the points of view represented and the functions to be performed by the advisory committee."[7] Discretionary committee agencies are required to develop a membership balance plan that describes how the agency will

[6]The five subcommittees were (1) food and nutrient intakes and health: current status and trends; (2) dietary patterns, foods and nutrients, and health outcomes; (3) diet and physical activity behavior change; (4) food and physical activity environments; and (5) food sustainability and safety. Working/writing groups were sodium, added sugars, saturated fats, and food and physical activity environments.

[7]Federal Advisory Committee Act, 1972, Public Law 92-463, 86 Stat 770, § 5(b)(2).

attain fairly balanced membership.[8] The membership balance plan is provided to the committee management secretariat as part of the required consultation process for establishing, renewing, or reestablishing a discretionary advisory committee. A membership balance plan can include elements such as points of view, other balance factors an agency identifies as important to achieve a balanced group, and the candidate identification process (GSA, 2011a). Although not required, a membership balance plan is also recommended for nondiscretionary advisory committees.

The points of view section in the 2015 DGAC restates the categories of expertise identified in the charter and underscores the point that members represent themselves and personal viewpoints, not those of a specific group. The plan lists other factors aimed to support balance including diversity across geographic areas, academic institutions, gender, race, ethnicity, and disability.

The membership balance plan for the 2015 DGAC describes a general candidate identification process, beginning with a notice in the *Federal Register*. Various offices within HHS and USDA review the nominees and identify qualified candidates, as well as those with the experience to potentially serve in leadership positions.[9] For the 2015 advisory committee, a list of primaries and alternates was developed and primaries were submitted through the formal nomination request to the secretaries of HHS and USDA (USDA/HHS, 2016a).

Bylaws

Federal advisory committees may operate in accordance with bylaws (also referred to as operating procedures). In addition to the committee's purpose, authority, membership selection, and appointment processes, the bylaws can delineate procedures for meetings, receipt of public comments, voting, role of board officials, expenses and reimbursement, and additional information. However, there currently is no standard template for the content of bylaws for federal advisory committees.

Bylaws were proposed by USDA and HHS and agreed upon by each DGAC. The bylaws governing the 2015 DGAC affirm that its operations are in accordance with FACA. Details are described, such as that meeting agendas will be approved by the designated federal officer and announced in the *Federal Register*; a quorum—defined as at least two-

[8]41 C.F.R. § 102-3.60.

[9]Specifically, the HHS Office of Disease Prevention and Health Promotion; the USDA Food, Nutrition, and Consumer Services' Center for Nutrition Policy and Promotion; and the USDA Research, Education, and Economics' Agricultural Research Service review and evaluate nominations.

thirds of the committee's members—must be present for meetings to be held; meetings related to substance will be open to the public (some meetings are administrative in nature, such as training on ethics and compliance with federal advisory committee rules); and that no closed meetings are planned. As one way to enhance transparency, written public comments to the advisory committee are all shared with the public through an online public comments database. Documentation of advisory committee deliberations are made publicly available. The bylaws state that decisions of the advisory committee are generally to be made through consensus but allow for formal voting if needed and outline processes to do so. Roles of the committee's chair and the co-executive secretaries are described. The document also details allowable expenses. Finally, it identifies the lead department's committee management officer as an additional source of guidance to ensure the advisory committee meets its objectives and to oversee the advisory committee's work (USDA/HHS, 2016a).

Charge

The DGAC is charged by HHS and USDA with reviewing the latest scientific evidence to inform revisions to the current guidance. DGACs are constituted for 2 year periods to complete their tasks and submit their findings to the secretaries of HHS and USDA in the form of scientific reports, which include technical recommendations and rationale but do not translate recommendations into policy.

In the case of the 2015 advisory committee, the charge was to review the 2010 guidelines and identify where new evidence would likely exist that may update existing guidance or suggest areas for new recommendations. The charge emphasizes systematic reviews and analyses of evidence published since the last advisory committee's deliberations. The 2015 advisory committee was also directed to place its primary emphasis on topics of public health importance for Americans ages 2 years and older (HHS/USDA, 2015, part C).

The charge can change between editions as needed. For example, the guidelines have historically focused on adults and children 2 years of age and older. However, the USDA-HHS Dietary Guidance Development Project for Pregnancy and Birth to 24 Months has initiated a project to develop advice for expanding the *DGA* beginning with the 2020–2025 edition (Raiten et al., 2014). Per the Agricultural Act of 2014, the guidelines will include pregnant women and children under the age of 2 years.

Public Comments Database

To promote transparency and public participation, the departments created an electronic database at www.dietaryguidelines.gov. This database is accessible to the public, as well as members of the advisory committee, and allows people to submit and access comments submitted for the committee's consideration. The comments are processed and organized by federal staff.

CURRENT ADVISORY COMMITTEE SELECTION PROCESS

The selection process is designed by HHS and USDA to vet the proposed slate within the departments, while also complying with FACA. Steps involved with the selection process include soliciting candidates, reviewing nomination packages and creating a slate of potential members, approving the nomination request package, and finally, formal appointment (see Figure 2-1). The nomination process begins while the aforementioned administrative tasks to establish the advisory committee are completed. The entire nomination process for the 2015 advisory committee took 7 months.

The co-executive secretaries initiate the process to form a federal advisory committee, which begins with announcing the intent to establish the advisory committee, solicitation of nominations, and formation of the charter. Nominees are solicited through a number of media, including the *Federal Register*, federal online mailing lists, and stakeholder communications. The *Federal Register* announcement of intent to establish the DGAC and solicitation of nominations lists the workplan (e.g., timing and number of meetings), general selection criteria, and categories of expertise sought. It also lists the information required to submit a nomination, including

1. a nomination letter and the qualifications of the nominee, as well as confirmation from the nominee that he or she would be willing to serve if asked;
2. nominee's contact information; and
3. curriculum vitae or resume, limited to no more than 10 pages.

The call for nominations for the 2015 DGAC lasted 45 days, resulting in 185 nominations (USDA/HHS, 2016b).

Initial reviews are conducted by the four co-executive secretaries who convene repeatedly to narrow the candidate pool to those who meet the requirements stated in the balance plan and charter. Remaining nominees are assessed for their abilities to contribute to the committee, both with respect to their specific areas of expertise as well as the breadth of their

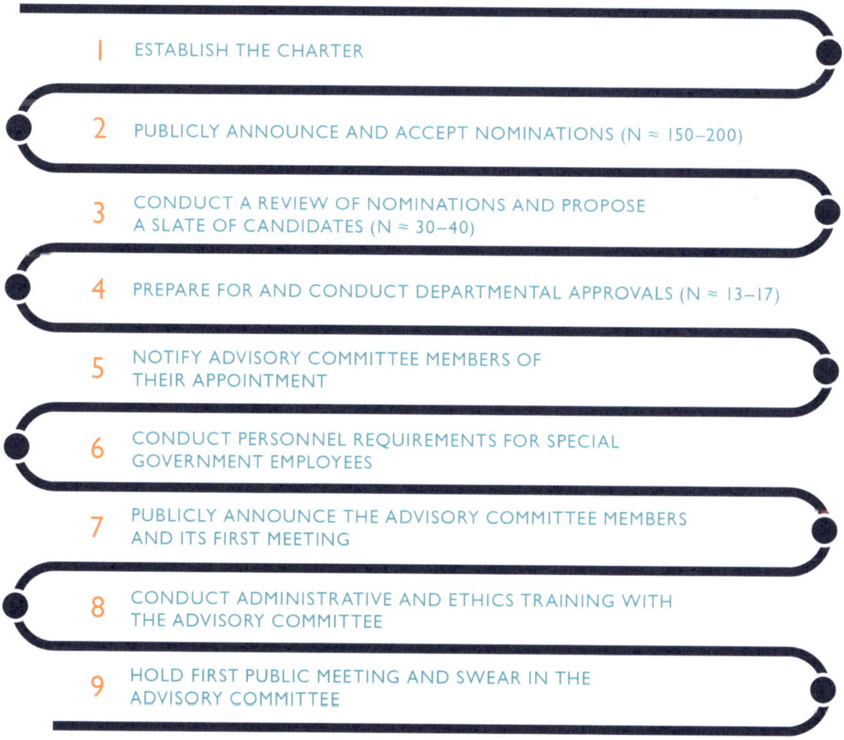
1 ESTABLISH THE CHARTER
2 PUBLICLY ANNOUNCE AND ACCEPT NOMINATIONS (N ≈ 150–200)
3 CONDUCT A REVIEW OF NOMINATIONS AND PROPOSE A SLATE OF CANDIDATES (N ≈ 30–40)
4 PREPARE FOR AND CONDUCT DEPARTMENTAL APPROVALS (N ≈ 13–17)
5 NOTIFY ADVISORY COMMITTEE MEMBERS OF THEIR APPOINTMENT
6 CONDUCT PERSONNEL REQUIREMENTS FOR SPECIAL GOVERNMENT EMPLOYEES
7 PUBLICLY ANNOUNCE THE ADVISORY COMMITTEE MEMBERS AND ITS FIRST MEETING
8 CONDUCT ADMINISTRATIVE AND ETHICS TRAINING WITH THE ADVISORY COMMITTEE
9 HOLD FIRST PUBLIC MEETING AND SWEAR IN THE ADVISORY COMMITTEE

FIGURE 2-1 Current process for selecting the Dietary Guidelines Advisory Committee.
NOTE: Total time for 2015 DGAC nominations process: 7 months.
SOURCE: Abstracted from USDA/HHS, 2016a.

experiences. Additionally, individuals' abilities to collaborate and work well with others, as well as skills related to communication and leadership, are considered. Members are selected to represent themselves and their own best judgment, not those of an employer or group. The candidates that collectively (1) reflect the requirements in the charter and membership balance plan and (2) address the advisory committee's charge are formed into a slate to be reviewed by the respective USDA and HHS offices. Feedback from the assistant secretary for health and the USDA undersecretaries of food, nutrition, and consumer services and research, education, and economics are passed back to the co-executive secretaries, and revisions are made as needed. Further vetting and consideration, including background checks, are conducted by the lead agency. The final slate is included with other materials, such as biographical sketches and decision memoranda, to form a nominations request package. The package is routed to the secretaries for their approval.

Advisory committee members are then notified of their appointments. However, substantive work cannot commence until members are sworn in during the first public meeting. In accordance with FACA, the members and first meeting details are published in the *Federal Register* at least 15 days prior to the meeting (USDA/HHS, 2016a).

The lead agency finalizes appointments as special government employees by ensuring that personnel actions and ethics requirements are met. This includes a disclosure of financial conflicts of interest (through Office of Government Ethics Form 450), reviewed by the lead agency. Members are finally required to undergo administrative training prior to their first meeting to review FACA, the charter and charge, and expectations of a special government employee.

DIETARY GUIDELINES ADVISORY COMMITTEE OPERATING PROCESS

Over their 30 year history, the DGACs have improved their processes for evaluating science. This evolution reflects updates in nutrition science and innovations in methods for developing public health guidance (USDA, 2016). For example, the Dietary Reference Intakes (DRIs) provide the infrastructure for the guidelines by establishing intake values and safe upper levels of nutrient consumption (IOM, 2003). A complete set of DRIs—recommended nutrient intakes—was not available for inclusion in the *DGA* until the 2005 edition (IOM, 2004). The stated philosophy of the *DGA* is that the recommendations should promote health with the ultimate goal of improving diets and decreasing risk of chronic disease by reducing inadequate or excessive intakes of food, nutrients, and calories. This goal is important to keep in mind as specific DRIs may be updated prior to or during the *2020–2025 DGA*. As updates occur, these developments in nutrition science will need to be taken into consideration by the DGAC. Similarly, the Nutrition Evidence Library (NEL) was created to bring tailored systematic reviews into the process. The 2010–2015 edition was the first *DGA* to use the NEL.

To provide background for the selection of members, the following section briefly describes how the DGAC operated in 2015 and how advisory committee members functioned. A more detailed description of the technical processes for evaluating the science will be provided in this National Academies committee's second report.

The charge to the advisory committee is to "examine the previous edition of the *DGA* and determine topics for which new scientific evidence is likely to be available that may inform revisions to the current guidance or suggest new guidance" (USDA/HHS, 2016a). To address its charge, the advisory committee breaks into topic-specific subcommittees, each of which is led by a chair; DGAC members are all expected to serve on multiple subcommittees. These subcommittees identify topics for consideration and develop research questions within each topic. Consultants can also be identified and invited by the DGAC to partake in subcommittee deliberations. While consultants receive training and are cleared through the federal process like the DGAC members, they are not members of the full committee (USDA/HHS, 2016c).

Next, the advisory committee determines the best approach to answer each question identified by the subcommittees, many of which may require a combination of methods to address. The 2010 and 2015 DGACs considered four types of evidence: (1) original systematic reviews commissioned by the DGAC with support from USDA's NEL, (2) systematic reviews or reports existing in the literature, (3) data analyses (e.g., intakes of foods and nutrients), and (4) food pattern modeling analyses. Other sources of information for the advisory committee to consider come from expert speakers and public comments. Through their discussions, the subcommittees assess the evidence and draft conclusions for consideration by the full DGAC (USDA/HHS, 2016c). The advisory committee works together to produce conclusions and draft the final report. Historically the *DGA* has been developed by consensus, but that decision is made by each DGAC itself.

CONCLUSION

In the development of the *DGA*, USDA and HHS convene a scientific advisory committee to evaluate the evidence and suggest updates to the previous edition. The DGAC has become a critical piece of the process to update the guidelines. This chapter described the process designed by the departments for selecting the advisory committee and its operating procedures, and the criteria the process must include to be in compliance with FACA.

REFERENCES

GAO (U.S. General Accounting Office). 1984. *National Academy of Sciences' reports on diet and health—are they credible and consistent?* GAO publication RCED-84-109. Washington, DC: U.S. General Accounting Office.

GSA (U.S. General Services Administration). 2011a. *Federal advisory committee membership balance plan* https://obamawhitehouse.archives.gov/sites/default/files/microsites/ostp/b_flaak_balance_plan.pdf (accessed October 5, 2017).

GSA. 2011b. *Preparing federal advisory committee charters.* https://www.gsa.gov/policy-regulations/policy/federal-advisory-committee-management/advice-and-guidance/federal-advisory-committee-charters (accessed October 5, 2017).

GSA. 2016. *GSA order: GSA Federal Advisory Committee Management Program.* ADM 5420.40E. Washington, DC. https://www.gsa.gov/portal/getMediaData?mediaId=139662 (accessed October 5, 2017).

HHS (U.S. Department of Health and Human Services). 1988. *The Surgeon General's report on nutrition and health.* DHHS publication PHS 88-50210. Washington, DC: U.S. Government Printing Office.

HHS/USDA (U.S. Department of Health and Human Services/U.S. Department of Agriculture). 2013 (unpublished). *History of dietary guidance development in the United States and the* Dietary Guidelines for Americans.

HHS/USDA. 2015. *Scientific Report of the 2015 Dietary Guidelines Advisory Committee.* Washington, DC: USDA, Agricultural Research Service.

IOM (Institute of Medicine). 1994. *How should the Recommended Dietary Allowances be revised?* Washington, DC: National Academy Press.

IOM. 2003. *Dietary Reference Intakes: Applications in dietary planning.* Washington, DC: The National Academies Press.

IOM. 2004. *Dietary Reference Intakes: Water, potassium, sodium, chloride, and sulfate.* Washington, DC: The National Academies Press.

NRC (National Research Council). 1989. *Diet and health: Implications for reducing chronic disease risk.* Washington, DC: National Academy Press.

OGE (U.S. Office of Government Ethics). 2016. *Advisory committee members.* https://www.oge.gov/Web/oge.nsf/Resources/Advisory+Committee+Members (accessed October 5, 2017).

Raiten, D. J., R. Raghavan, A. Porter, J. E. Obbagy, and J. M. Spahn. 2014. Executive summary: Evaluating the evidence base to support the inclusion of infants and children from birth to 24 mo of age in the *Dietary Guidelines for Americans*—"the B-24 project." *American Journal of Clinical Nutrition* 99(3):663s-691s.

Secretary of Health and Human Services. 2013. *Charter: 2015 v.* Washington, DC. https://health.gov/dietaryguidelines/dgac2015-charter-final.pdf (accessed October 5, 2017).

USDA (U.S. Department of Agriculture). 2016 (unpublished). *Understanding the committee's charge: A discussion with the sponsor.* Presentation to the Committee to Review the Process to Update the *Dietary Guidelines for Americans.*

USDA/HHS (U.S. Department of Agriculture/U.S. Department of Health and Human Services). 2016a (unpublished). Dietary Guidelines for Americans: *Process brief, sections 1–3.* Prepared for the Committee to Review the Process to Update the *Dietary Guidelines for Americans.*

USDA/HHS. 2016b (unpublished). *HMD follow-up questions for USDA.* Response to Committee to Review the Process to Update the *Dietary Guidelines for Americans.*

USDA/HHS. 2016c (unpublished). Dietary Guidelines for Americans: *Process brief, sections 4–5.* Prepared for the Committee to Review the Process to Update the *Dietary Guidelines for Americans.*

3

Models for Composing an Advisory Committee

The members selected to serve on an advisory committee can affect the integrity, perception, credibility, and acceptance of the work performed. Membership selection, therefore, is a critical initial step in the overall process. In general, an agency or organization that convenes an advisory committee has the authority to decide how the members are identified, screened, vetted, and appointed. This has led to the implementation of a variety of approaches. Some of the differences are institutional, as not all convening entities have the infrastructure or resources needed to execute the same protocol. The specific committee's function can also be a source of variability. Committees with charges that differ in scope and intended audiences may use different techniques to optimize the composition of membership. Because the wide variety of methods, purposes, and outcomes makes it challenging to conduct systematic evaluations of best practices, this National Academies of Sciences, Engineering, and Medicine (the National Academies) committee was not able to identify a set of best practices. Instead, it found that the heterogeneity offers a range of options to consider for enhancing the Dietary Guidelines Advisory Committee (DGAC) selection process.

Determining the usefulness of alternative committee selection approaches is challenging, as the applicability of a specific process is circumstantial. To contextualize the approach used to select members to the DGAC and to consider opportunities for improvement, this National Academies committee explored different membership selection processes across a variety of disciplines and organizations. The analysis contained in this chapter exclusively highlights examples of committees whose processes differ from those used to select the DGAC. Committees whose processes are similar to the DGAC are purposely not discussed in this report. The sections that follow summarize key differences in advisory committee selection processes. Inclusion of a selection process herein does not reflect this National Academies committee's endorsement, but rather describes an environmental scan of the variability and options that exist.

VARIOUS SELECTION PROCESSES USED FOR FEDERAL ADVISORY COMMITTEES

Federal advisory committees are underpinned by the same key legislation, namely the Federal Advisory Committee Act (FACA), which governs the establishment, operation, oversight, and termination of advisory committees within the executive branch of the federal government (see Chapter 2 for additional details). Because each agency is required to develop its own administrative procedures describing how it will implement FACA while being consistent with the law and the 2001 Final Rule, an assessment of other federal advisory committees offers insight into processes that are considered permissible under the same general confines.

This National Academies committee used the FACA database and a review of other reports to search for federal advisory committees with unique selection processes that were also different from the process used for the DGAC (CRS, 2007; GAO, 2004; GSA, 2016). Advisory committees that were current, chartered, and active across a range of agencies were considered. With approximately 1,000 federal advisory committees active at a given time, this committee was unable to comprehensively explore the breadth of all possibilities. This assessment, therefore, was not intended to be systematic or exhaustive, but rather exploratory, to help identify components of the selection process that could be adapted or modified to enhance the transparency, minimize bias, and incorporate a range of viewpoints and expertise into future DGACs.

The DGAC selection process was compared to the 11 illustrative examples listed in Table 3-1. An initial review of the FACA database and reports from the U.S. Government Accountability Office and the General Services Administration were used to identify federal advisory committees with innovative and unique processes related to the selection of members. These examples were selected for their procedural differences from the DGAC process related to membership designations; methods for soliciting nominations; and the steps taken to screen, vet, and appoint members. Specific details were identified in the committees' charters, membership balance plans, websites, and *Federal Register* notices. This National Academies committee recognizes that processes are more

TABLE 3-1 Federal Advisory Committees Chosen to Illustrate Variability in Membership Selection Processes

Advisory Committee	Sponsoring Agency	Individual or Entity Being Advised
Discretionary		
Advisory Committee on Agriculture Statistics (ACAS)	USDA	• Secretary, Agriculture
Chemical Safety Advisory Committee (CSAC)	EPA	• Office of Pollution Prevention and Toxics
FDIC Advisory Committee on Economic Inclusion (FDIC ComE-IN)	FDIC	• Chairman of the Board of Directors, FDIC
Homeland Security Information Network Advisory Committee (HSINAC)	DHS	• DHS Leadership
National Advisory Committee on Racial, Ethnic, Other Populations (NAC-REOP)	DOC	• Director, Census Bureau
Nondiscretionary		
Advisory Board on Toxic Substances and Worker Health (ABTSWH)	DOL	• Secretary, Labor
Arthritis Advisory Committee (AAC)	HHS	• Commissioner, FDA
Health IT Policy Committee (HITPC)	HHS	• National Coordinator for Health IT
Healthcare Infection Control Practices Advisory Committee (HICPAC)	HHS	• Secretary, HHS • Director, CDC • Deputy Director, Office of Infectious Diseases, CDC • Director, National Center for Emerging and Zoonotic Infectious Diseases (NCEZID), CDC • Director, Division of Healthcare Quality Promotion (DHQP), NCEZID, CDC
National Vaccine Advisory Committee (NVAC)	HHS	• Director of the National Vaccine Program (Assistant Secretary for Health)
Physician-Focused Payment Model Technical Advisory Committee (PTAC)	HHS	• Secretary, HHS

NOTE: CDC = Centers for Disease Control and Prevention; U.S. DHS = U.S. Department of Homeland Security; DOC = U.S. Department of Commerce; DOL = U.S. Department of Labor; EPA = U.S. Environmental Protection Agency; FDA = U.S. Food and Drug Administration; FDIC = Federal Deposit Insurance Corporation; HHS = U.S. Department of Health and Human Services; IT = information technology; USDA = U.S. Department of Agriculture.

involved and nuanced than what can be provided for in descriptive summaries, and that sponsoring agencies may deviate from what is initially planned. This assessment, however, must assume agencies fully implement the procedures as outlined. The DGAC procedures included in this section are discussed in more detail in Chapter 2. Detail extending beyond what was included in previous charters and membership balance plans are included, but are noted as such. Across the illustrative examples, key differences were noted in types of members sought, the process for soliciting nominees, and the review of candidates and appointments.

Advisory Committee Composition—Membership Designation

As part of the chartering process, sponsoring agencies are asked to provide a description of how members will be designated. Federal advisory committee members can be designated as a special government employee, representative, regular government employee, or ex officio members. Some advisory committees have also made use of nonvoting members, including those considered ex officio, industry representatives, and liaisons to special interest groups. A member's designation indicates the perspective he or she is expected to bring to the advisory committee (i.e., individual or representing a particular bias). The designation may have implications for which ethical standards and laws regarding conflicts of interest are applicable. Importantly, as noted in Box 2-2, representative members are not subject to criminal financial conflict of interest laws, while all other members are. Another difference among membership designations is that members may be eligible to receive compensation for their work if approved by appointing authority, while employees and officers of the federal government are not eligible.

The DGAC includes only special government employees, which was found not to be an uncommon practice. However, the illustrative examples demonstrate that there is no single approach to composing an advisory committee, with respect to membership designation, and that some committees use a blend of special government employees, representatives, regular government employees, and ex officio members (see Table 3-2).

Solicitations for Nominations

Sponsoring agencies can describe how candidates will be identified in the membership balance plan, which is required for discretionary committees and encouraged for nondiscretionary committees. Although dependent on the structure and function of the advisory committee, agencies tend to seek nominations from a range of individuals and groups including, but not limited to, professional, scientific, and medical societies and organizations; stakeholder and advocacy groups; current and former committee members; and relevant federal agencies or staff. One approach to announcing the public call for nominations, common across the illustrative examples, is publishing a notice in the *Federal Register*. The notices can include information about the advisory committee (e.g., authority, purpose) and about how nominations can be submitted. Other dissemination channels are also used. The Advisory Board on Toxic Substances and Worker Health, for instance, planned to use "existing outreach tools, such as email groups and social media tools, to publicize vacancies and identify as many potential candidates as possible" (DOL, 2015d).

The materials collected during the initial phase of advisory committee formations have implications for the screening of nominees. For example, some sponsoring agencies will only consider individuals with complete applications. As presented in Table 3-3, there are common items requested, such as the nominee's curriculum vitae or résumé, but no standard set of materials is used across agencies or advisory committees.

Evidence from the illustrative examples indicates that sponsoring agencies have the ability to tailor their nomination solicitation approach. The extent to which agencies receive input and guidance on their customized strategy is not well characterized. One example, however, was identified. The membership balance plan for the Chemical Safety Advisory Committee, which is convened by the U.S. Environmental Protection Agency (EPA), noted that the designated federal officer was to consult with EPA's Office of Diversity, Advisory Committee Management and Outreach, to develop an approved outreach plan for identifying committee members (EPA, 2015d). This National Academies committee could not identify an oversight step of the nomination process in its review of the other illustrative examples.

Although this National Academies committee was unable to assess the effectiveness of different nomination solicitation models (e.g., reach of announcement, nomination information, transparency), it did identify one example of enhanced transparency. As outlined in a 2015 *Federal Register* notice, nominations for the Chemical Safety Advisory Committee (CSAC) could be delivered by hand, sent by mail, or submitted through the Federal eRulemaking Portal (EPA, 2015b).[1] Nominations capture the name of the commenter and the materials submitted, and they are openly available online for review (EPA, 2015c). Across the illustrative examples, this was the only federal advisory committee in which nominees were recorded in a publicly accessible platform.

[1]The Federal eRulemaking Portal can be found at www.regulations.gov (accessed October 24, 2017).

TABLE 3-2 Membership Designations for Select Federal Advisory Committees

	Discretionary						Nondiscretionary				
	DGAC	ACAS	CSAC	FDIC ComE-IN	HSINAC	NAC-REOP	AAC	ABTSWH	HICPAC	HITPC	NVAC
Special government employee	X	X[a]	X		X	X	X[b]	X	X	X[a]	X
Representative		X		X		X				X[c]	X
Regular government employee			X		X		X			X[c]	
Ex officio		X[d]						X		X[c]	X[e]
Nonvoting member(s)							X[f]		X[g]		X[h]

NOTES: An X indicates the member type was described in the advisory committee's charter, balance plan, or other associated materials. A blank indicates such a member was not explicitly permitted or anticipated. Members of the Physician-Focused Payment Model Technical Advisory Committee (PTAC) "have been determined to be neither employees of the executive branch of the federal government nor 'special government employees'" (HHS, 2016c). As such, PTAC is not included in this table.

AAC = Arthritis Advisory Committee; ABTSWH = Advisory Board on Toxic Substances and Workers Health; ACAS = Advisory Committee on Agricultural Statistics; CSAC = Chemical Safety Advisory Committee; DGAC = Dietary Guidelines Advisory Committee; FACA = Federal Advisory Committee Act; FDIC = Federal Deposit Insurance Corporation; FDIC-ComE-IN = FDIC Advisory Committee on Economic Inclusion; HICPAC = Healthcare Infection Control Practices Advisory Committee; HITPC = Health Information Technology Policy Committee; HSINAC = Homeland Security Information Network Advisory Committee; NAC-REOP = National Advisory Committee on Racial, Ethnic, and Other Populations; NVAC = National Vaccine Advisory Committee.

[a]The charter includes language about inclusion of special government employees, but none of the members in the FACA database for this committee are currently or have historically been designated as such.

[b]May include one technical qualified individual who identifies with consumer interests and is nominated by a consortium of consumer-oriented organizations.

[c]Based on search of current and historical membership in the FACA database. From 2009 through 2011, committee membership included regular government employees. Thereafter, all members were designated as either representative or ex officio.

[d]Voting status of the ex officio members is not specified in the charter.

[e]Ex officio members are nonvoting members.

[f]May include one nonvoting industry representative.

[g]Includes federal representatives and liaison representatives from a range of associations and stakeholder groups.

[h]Nonvoting members include those designated ex officio and liaison representatives of organizations and interest groups.

SOURCES: DOC, 2016a; DOL, 2015a; EPA, 2015a; FDIC, 2014; HHS, 2009, 2015a,b,e, 2016a,c; USDA, 2016a.

TABLE 3-3 Materials Requested to Nominate an Individual to Serve on Select Federal Advisory Committees

	Discretionary					Nondiscretionary					
	DGAC	ACAS	CSAC	HSINAC	NAC-REOP	AAC	ABTSWH	HICPAC	HITPC[a]	NVAC	PTAC
Letter of nomination	X				X					X	X
Letter(s) of recommendation						X[b]		X[c]	X[d]		
Statement from nominee	X			X		X[b]	X[e]			X	
Nominator's contact information	X									X	
Nominee's contact information	X					X	X[f]	X	X		
Nominee's curriculum vitae or résumé	X[g]			X[h]	X	X	X	X	X	X	X
Nominee's short biography									X		
Summary of nominee's qualifications							X[i]				
Membership background information form		X[j]									
Articles authored by nominee							X				
Nominee's active participation in organizations						X[b,k]					
Nominee's familiarity with the program							X[l]				
Completed OGE Form 450[m]				X							
Not specified			X								

NOTES: An X indicates the material was requested of a nominator, while a blank indicates the material was not specifically requested. This National Academies committee did not find evidence of a call for nominations for the FDIC Advisory Committee on Economic Inclusion, and as such it has been omitted from the table

AAC = Arthritis Advisory Committee; ABTSWH = Advisory Board on Toxic Substances and Workers Health; ACAS = Advisory Committee on Agricultural Statistics; CSAC = Chemical Safety Advisory Committee; DGAC = Dietary Guidelines Advisory Committee; FDA = U.S. Food and Drug Administration; FDIC = Federal Deposit Insurance Corporation; HICPAC; Healthcare Infection Control Practices Advisory Committee; HITPC = Health Information Technology Policy Committee; HSINAC = Homeland Security Information Network Advisory Committee; NAC-REOP = National Advisory Committee on Racial, Ethnic, and Other Populations; NVAC = National Vaccine Advisory Committee; OGE = Office of Government Ethics; PTAC = Physician-Focused Payment Model Technical Advisory Committee.

[a]Only accepts applications directly from the candidate.

[b]These materials are requested in the FDA Advisory Committee Membership Nomination Portal, but not explicitly requested in the *Federal Register* notice.

[c]At least one letter of recommendation must come from someone outside of the U.S. Department of Health and Human Services.

[d]Two letters of support are required.

[e]Nominees must acknowledge they are aware of their nomination, consent to having their name published in the *Federal Register*, are willing to actively participate, and verify they have no financial conflicts of interest.

[f]Includes the nominee's current employment or position.

[g]Limited to 10 pages or less.

[h]Limited to 2 pages or less.

[i]Nominators are also asked to specify which membership category the nominee is suited to represent.

[j]Candidates are asked to complete Form AD-755, "Advisory Committee or Research and Promotion Background Information." The form requests the individual to report his or her contact information, demographic characteristics (optional), current employment, specific expertise, affiliations with organizations, and sources of income other than primary employment.

[k]Only requested for individuals seeking a consumer representative appointment.

[l]The Advisory Board on Toxic Substances and Worker Health provides guidance on claims under the Energy Employee Occupational Illness Program Act (EEOIPA) program. The request for nominations asks for information about the nominee's experience with the EEOIPA program or one as technically complex.

[m]OGE Form 450 is a confidential financial disclosure form that asks filers to report their assets and income; liabilities; outside positions; agreements and arrangements; and gifts and travel reimbursements from the previous 12 months. Assets, income, and liabilities of the spouse and any dependent children must also be reported.

SOURCES: DHS, 2011; DOC, 2016b; DOL, 2015c; EPA, 2015b,c; FDA, 2016; GAO, 2015; HHS, 2014a,b, 2015c,g, 2016d; HHS/USDA, 2012; NASS, 2016.

Review of Candidates and Appointments

FACA does not stipulate how members should be appointed to federal advisory committees. Instead, the head of the agency establishing the federal advisory committee has the sole authority in appointing members, unless otherwise provided for in statute, presidential directive, or other establishment authority.[2] Agency heads are also responsible for ensuring the interests and affiliations of advisory committee members are reviewed for conformance with applicable conflict-of-interest statutes and other federal ethics rules.[3] Materials reviewed describing the 11 illustrative examples varied in their level of detail concerning agency-specific processes. Differences were identified in how nominees are initially screened, how candidates are vetted, and who has the authority to appoint members. Although screening and vetting are not always operationalized as distinct procedures, this National Academies committee uses the terms to connote two aspects of the selection processes. *Screening* is used to describe the initial appraisal of nominees' qualifications, generally in relation to their expertise unless otherwise noted. *Vetting* is used to describe a more comprehensive or thorough investigation into the candidates' background, including their affiliations, personal biases, personal and imputed financial conflicts of interest, and nonfinancial conflicts of interest (see Box 3-1).

Initial Screening of Nominees

Five of the illustrative examples described a preliminary screening of the nominees, prior to conducting an extensive background investigation or selecting a slate for final approvals. The designated federal officer and/or a team of program staffers were responsible for this initial narrowing of the candidate pool (see Table 3-4). Across the examples, screening generally involved an assessment of relatively subjective characteristics, such as expertise and leadership qualities. For the CSAC nominees, EPA also noted considering financial conflicts of interests and impartiality during this preliminary screening stage. The other illustrative examples described evaluating conflicts of interest later in the appointment process, if described at all (see "Vetting of Candidates" section). One unique process was noted for the National Vaccine Advisory Committee. The director of the National Vaccine Program is required to consult with the National Academy of Sciences (NAS) to determine if the candidates are qualified based on the criteria outlined in the *Federal Register* notice. This

---

[2] 41 C.F.R. § 102-3.130.

[3] 41 C.F.R. § 102-3.105.

is the only federal advisory committee this National Academies committee reviewed that uses a nongovernment entity to participate in the screening of nominees.

Vetting of Candidates

Vetting refers to a thorough review of candidates' backgrounds. Vetting procedures are often cited as a means for assessing candidates' biases and conflicts of interest (see Box 3-1).

As presented in Table 3-5, the illustrative examples have taken different approaches to vetting candidates. One broad approach is to seek approval of several offices or various positions within the agency. This presumably allows for the slate of candidates to be considered from individuals who may offer different perspectives. Other vetting procedures are specific to the appraisal of conflicts and other ethical considerations. These have included background checks and financial disclosures. While most of the vetting procedures are described as taking place after a slate of candidates is selected, the CSAC described considering financial conflicts and lack of impartiality as considerations that inform the development of the slate.

Assessment of financial conflicts of interest is at the forefront of the vetting of special and regular government employee candidates. Officers or employees of the executive branch of the U.S. government (which includes those designated as special government employees) may be charged under criminal law for participating in any government matter in which they have a financial interest. The federal U.S. Office of Government Ethics (OGE) provides overarching guidance for how executive branch agencies prevent conflicts of interest. Included are tools for identifying and managing conflicts of interest of those who serve on federal advisory committees (OGE, 2000). Based on an assessment of the regular government employee's position, rate of pay, and the regulations put forth by OGE, the appointee may be required to complete either an OGE Form 450 (Confidential Financial Disclosure Report; see Box 3-2) or OGE Form 278 (Public Financial Disclosure Report), in order for the agency to assess the potential for personal and imputed financial conflicts of interest.[4] Appointees designated as special government employees typically complete OGE Form 450. However, alternative procedures may be used in lieu of filing OGE Form 450.[5] Information submitted on OGE Form 450 is confidential and

[4]Imputed interests includes those of the candidate's spouse, minor child, general partner, outside employer, and persons or organizations with whom the candidate is negotiating or has an arrangement for employment.

[5]5 C.F.R. § 2634.905.

TABLE 3-4 Initial Screening of Nominees for Select Federal Advisory Committees

	Discretionary			Nondiscretionary		
	DGAC	CSAC	NAC-REOP	AAC	HICPAC	NVAC
Process	• Program staff at HHS and USDA[a] review nominees for their scientific expertise and leadership potential and create a primary and alternate slate of candidates	• Pool of nominees is reviewed to determine the need for additional outreach • Nominees are screened for financial conflicts of interest and appearance of lack of impartiality • Designated federal officer drafts list of candidates and alternates	• Designated federal officer, committee liaison officer, and internal team draft a list of "best-qualified"[b] candidates	• Designated federal officers and office/division directors are responsible for reviewing nominees for competence and suitability, including assessing alignment of background education, and experience with the function of the advisory committee; scientific and technical expertise; and leadership qualities	• Designated federal officer develops a candidate list	• Nominees are reviewed by senior-level management and program staff and sent to the National Academy of Sciences[c] • The National Academy of Sciences reviews nominees' qualifications and selects qualified candidates[d]

NOTES: The following committees were omitted from this table because a description of how the nominee pool was narrowed was not included in their charter or membership balance plan: Advisory Board on Toxic Substances and Worker Health, Advisory Committee on Agriculture Statistics, Federal Deposit Insurance Corporation Advisory Committee on Economic Inclusion, Health IT Policy Committee, Homeland Security Information Network Advisory Committee, and Physician-Focused Payment Model Technical Advisory Committee.
AAC = Arthritis Advisory Committee; CSAC = Chemical Safety Advisory Committee; DGAC = Dietary Guidelines Advisory Committee; HHS = U.S. Department of Health and Human Services; HICPAC; Healthcare Infection Control Practices Advisory Committee; HITPC = Health Information Technology Policy Committee; NAC-REOP = National Advisory Committee on Racial, Ethnic, and Other Populations; NVAC = National Vaccine Advisory Committee; USDA = U.S. Department of Agriculture.

[a]In recent revisions, the program staff have been the co-executive secretaries appointed by Office of Disease Prevention and Health Promotion (HHS); Food, Nutrition, and Consumer Services Center for Nutrition Research (USDA); and the Research, Education, and Economics Agricultural Research Service (USDA). See Chapter 2 for additional details.

[b]Term used in the 2016 membership balance plan.

[c]As described in the 2015 membership balance plan.

[d]Under 42 U.S.C. § 300aa-5, the director of the National Vaccine Program appoints NVAC committee members in consultation with the National Academy of Sciences.

SOURCES: DOC, 2012; EPA, 2015d; HHS, 2015d,f, 2016b; USDA/HHS, 2016.

TABLE 3-5 Process Used to Vet Candidates for Select Federal Advisory Committees

Discretionary				Nondiscretionary			
DGAC	ACAS	CSAC	NAC-REOP[e]	AAC	ABTSWH	HICPAC	NVAC
• HHS Assistant Secretary for Health and USDA Undersecretary of FNCS and REE review and approve the proposed slate[a] • Reviewed by the office responsible for committee management • Senior-level officials review candidates' qualifications[b]	• Candidates' names and information are submitted to the USDA White House liaison's office for vetting, which includes a background check[c]	• SGE candidates are researched to determine whether they are a federally registered lobbyist • Nominees are screened for financial conflicts of interest and appearance of lack of impartiality[d]	• An internal vet through the sponsoring agency • A Lexis-Nexis check • An ethics check[f] • Verification the candidate is not a registered foreign agent or a registered lobbyist • Security clearance or assurance paperwork • Financial disclosure (OGE Form 450), for members to be appointed as SGEs	• Candidate's curriculum vitae, conflict-of-interest form, publication list, and committee affiliations are reviewed[g]	• The names and affiliations of potential members are published in the *Federal Register* and feedback from interested parties is sought	• Candidates are contacted for interest and availability and are reviewed by the director of the NCEZID • Candidate list is then submitted to the Management Analysis Services Office (CDC) and the Office of the Director (CDC)	• Candidates' information is forwarded to the department committee management office for the necessary review[h]

NOTES: The following committees were omitted from this table because a description of how the candidates were vetted was not included in their charter or membership balance plan: Arthritis Advisory Committee; Federal Deposit Insurance Corporation Advisory Committee on Economic Inclusion; Health Information Technology Policy Committee; Homeland Security Information Network Advisory Committee; National Advisory Committee on Racial, Ethnic, and Other Populations; and Physician-Focused Payment Model Technical Advisory Committee.

AAC = Arthritis Advisory Committee; ABTSWH = Advisory Board on Toxic Substances and Workers Health; ACAS = Advisory Committee on Agricultural Statistics; CDC = Centers for Disease Control and Prevention; CSAC = Chemical Safety Advisory Committee; DGAC = Dietary Guidelines Advisory Committee; FACA = Federal Advisory Committee Act; FNCS = Food, Nutrition, and Consumer Services; HHS = U.S. Department of Health and Human Services; HICPAC = Healthcare Infection Control Practices Advisory Committee; NAC-REOP = National Advisory Committee on Racial, Ethnic, and Other Populations; NCEZID = National Center for Emerging and Zoonotic Infectious Diseases (CDC); NVAC = National Vaccine Advisory Committee; OGE = Office of Government Ethics; REE = Research, Education, and Economics; SGE = special government employee; USDA = U.S. Department of Agriculture.

[a]The proposed slate is compiled after two stages of screening. The initial screening identifies potentially qualified candidates, based on the criteria listed in the charter. This smaller pool is further narrowed by considering a range of factors, including potential intellectual conflicts of interest.

[b]Vetting by senior-level officials includes comprehensive personal and professional background checks, which encompasses but is not limited to an assessment of the candidate's criminal history, affiliations and associations, and prior involvement with the department.

[c]Background checks are used to assess whether candidates have a conflict of interest that would rise to the level of a criminal or ethical violation, and therefore disqualify them from serving on the advisory committee.

[d]This process was also included in Table 3-4, describing the initial screening of nominees.

[e]NAC-REOP uses the FACA membership process outlined by the Office of the General Counsel of the U.S. Department of Commerce.

[f]Described as ensuring "that members do not represent organizations that appear on the secretary's disqualification statement, if appointed by the secretary" (DOC, 2015).

[g]Used in the assessment of committee members' point of view and overall committee balance.

[h]Used in the final determination whether the candidate is sufficiently qualified to be appointed to the advisory committee.

SOURCES: DOC, 2012, 2015; DOL, 2015d; EPA, 2015d; HHS, 2015d,f; USDA, 2016b; USDA/HHS, 2016.

BOX 3-1
Defining Bias and Conflict of Interest

Although they are often considered together, bias and conflict of interest are distinct. This National Academies committee considers a bias to be an intellectual predisposition toward a particular perspective and an inherent part of being a subject-matter expert. Because bias is intrinsically subjective, it is difficult to identify and measure (Jacobson, 2016). Given this, an advisory committee requiring specific expertise to address its charge cannot be entirely free of biases. Biases are, therefore, something to be managed rather than eliminated.

Conflicts of interest, in contrast, are "a set of circumstances that creates a risk that professional judgment or actions regarding a primary interest will be unduly influenced by a secondary interest" (IOM, 2009). Individuals can be influenced by factors that are financial and nonfinancial in nature.

Assessing conflicts of interest does not mean that an individual's behavior is unethical. Instead, it is intended to identify an unacceptable risk of undue influence. Policies covering conflicts of interest generally do not presume that financial gains or other conflicts necessarily sway an individual's viewpoints (IOM, 2009). Nonfinancial conflicts of interest can be just as, if not more, influential than financial conflicts (Akl et al., 2014; Bero, 2014; Guyatt et al., 2010; IOM, 2009). Additionally, while there is a difference between actual and perceived conflicts, the perception is sometimes enough to promote mistrust.

cannot be released, even through a Freedom of Information Act request. Special government employees serving on federal advisory committees may be granted a waiver if it is determined that the need for their service outweighs the potential conflict.[6]

Capturing and evaluating biases and nonfinancial conflicts of interest poses a challenge for any organization convening a committee (GAO, 2004) (see Box 3-3). Indeed, this is reflected in the illustrative examples, which did not provide extensive descriptions of such assessments. One example for capturing nonfinancial conflicts was identified. EPA has adapted the standard confidential financial disclosure form for special government employees and added Section 6, which includes supplemental ethics questions for the potential committee member to complete (EPA, 2016). Questions ask the candidate to report anything that would be perceived as jeopardizing their impartiality, whether they had been involved in any of the documents that will be reviewed, what other committees on which they have served, and if they have made any public comments

[6]18 U.S.C. § 208(b)(3).

BOX 3-2
Financial Conflicts of Interest Reported on OGE Form 450

The reporting period for OGE Form 450 is the 12 months preceding filing. The individual is asked to declare assets and income for themselves, spouse, and/or dependent children. Special government employees, unlike regular government employees, are not asked to declare gifts and travel reimbursements. Financial information is declared and collected in the following reporting categories, including examples of each:

- *Assets and income*, such as salary, stocks, bonds, trust holdings, real estate, honoraria greater than $200
- *Liabilities (debts)*, such as liability or personal loan more than $10,000 other than a loan from a financial institution or business entity
- *Outside positions*, such as officer, director, employee, trustee, or consultant of any of the following: corporation, partnership, trust, or other business entity; nonprofit or volunteer organization; educational institution
- *Agreements or arrangements*, such as continuing pension or benefit plan maintained by a former employer, a leave of absence, future employment, severance payments
- *Gifts and travel reimbursements*, such as lodging, transportation or food totaling more than $375 from any one source; any gifts totaling more than $375 from any one source

SOURCE: OGE, 2015.

on the topics under consideration. While the burden of disclosure remains on the individual candidate, EPA Form 3110-48 represents one approach to documenting and assessing biases and nonfinancial conflicts of interest.

The vetting process is not restricted to background investigations conducted by the agency. One example incorporated public feedback as part of the vetting process. A 2015 *Federal Register* notice listed the names, credentials, and affiliations of each candidate for the Advisory Board on Toxic Substances and Worker Health, and gave the public 14 days to provide comment before final appointments were made (DOL, 2015b). Public comment on the list of candidates, however, was not a process seen in any of the other illustrative examples.

The presence of conflicts of interest is not always an automatic disqualifier. Members of the Physician-Focused Payment Model Technical Advisory Committee (PTAC), for example, operate under bylaws that explicitly outline how conflicts of interest will be managed (HHS, 2016c). The legislation authorizing the formation of the PTAC states that for the

BOX 3-3
Assessing Biases and Nonfinancial Conflicts of Interest

Nonfinancial conflicts, biases, and perspectives are difficult to capture and evaluate, as they tend to be subjective in nature. Sometimes they can be identified through a review of previously published positions or statements. Other times, they can only be revealed through conversations with the individual, which also assumes the person is being truthful. Because there are no objective or definitive measures, biases and nonfinancial conflicts of interests can be easily overlooked.

This National Academies committee's review of the published literature suggests a range of different types of nonfinancial conflicts of interest exists (AHRQ, 2015; Boyd and Bero, 2006; Boyd et al., 2012; Guyatt et al., 2010; NHMRC, 2012), including

- *Intellectual*, such as entrenched opinions, passions, public statements relating to potential recommendations
- *Organizational or institutional affiliations*, such as testimony, speeches, participation in advocacy or interest groups
- *Advisory roles*, such as scientific or technical advisory boards or committees
- *Academic or professional commitments*, such as leadership roles, fellowships
- *Academic or professional advancement*, such as recognition, promotion
- *Research and/or publications*, such as grants received, authorship of research and/or publications directly related to the subject
- *Individual beliefs and values*, such as political, ideological, religious, cultural

Across the published reports, no differences were observed in the reporting period for financial versus nonfinancial conflicts of interest; however, in the case of nonfinancial conflicts, such as intellectual bias or individual beliefs that can be longstanding, timing may not be relevant. The implications of the particular committee's work speak to the challenges of identifying potential conflicts. An organizational affiliation, for example, may not be an immediately apparent conflict, but it may require determination of potential policy implications or advocacy outcomes of the recommendations to consider whether it constitutes a conflict.

purposes of filing financial disclosures, members are treated as employees of Congress. This means that members are not classified as special government employees and are not subject to the same rules regarding conflicts of interest and ethical standards. Instead, each committee member is responsible for disclosing at the beginning of each meeting any involvement with the materials to be discussed. It is then up to the other members of the advisory committee to collectively decide the extent to which the potentially conflicted member may participate in the meeting. Both the potential conflict and the advisory committee's decision on the member's involvement in the discussions and voting on the topic are disclosed to the public. This model engages members in managing conflict of interest and promotes transparency.

Appointment Authorities

Unless directed otherwise by statute or presidential directive, the head of the agency establishing the federal advisory committee has the sole authority to appoint federal advisory committee members. Mandates have been put forth assigning appointing authority to political appointees and other leaders. For example, members of the nondiscretionary Health IT Policy Committee are appointed by the secretary of health and human services (3 members); the majority leader of the Senate (1 member); the minority leader of the Senate (1 member); the majority lead of the House of Representatives (1 member); the minority leader of the House of Representatives (1 member); the Comptroller General of the United States (13 members); and the President (relevant representative members) (HHS, 2009).

Committees That Operate Under Section 15 of the Federal Advisory Committee Act

Section 15 of FACA mandates specific procedures for committees appointed by the NAS and the National Academy of Public Administration that provide advice to a federal agency under an agreement with it. Section 15 requires the two academies to "provide public notice of the names and brief biographies of individuals that the Academy appoints or intends to appoint to serve on the committee" and to "provide a reasonable opportunity for the public to comment on such appointments before they are made."[7] This requirement is in contrast to the noted procedures for federal advisory committees that operate under the other provisions of FACA.

SELECTION PROCESSES USED FOR NON-FACA COMMITTEES

Other selection approaches are used by groups that do not operate under FACA. This National Academies committee explored the processes of organizations whose recommendations, guidelines, and policies have national or international implications. Many convening entities that do not operate under FACA publish documentation of their processes by posting procedure manuals online or publishing the information as jour-

[7]Federal Advisory Committee Act Amendments of 1997, § 15(b)(1).

nal articles. There is no standard set of information that must be included in such descriptions, making it almost impossible to assess and compare processes. Furthermore, there is no central repository of the different processes, as there is with federal advisory committees. As such, this National Academies committee was limited in its ability to comprehensively explore the range of processes used to compose non-FACA committees. This appraisal, therefore, is not intended to be exhaustive. The procedures to select non-FACA committee members largely differed from federal advisory committees with respect to documenting how financial and nonfinancial conflicts of interest are identified and managed. Based on a review of the literature and the experiences of this National Academies committee, a large number of governmental and nongovernmental organizations—both domestic and international—were studied. The processes developed by governmental organizations tended to be more transparent and have more explicit rules to follow than nongovernmental organizations. Five examples with unique conflict of interest procedures are described below.

U.S. Preventive Services Task Force

The U.S. Preventive Services Task Force (USPSTF) is an independent committee that makes evidence-based recommendations about health promotion and clinical preventative services in the primary care setting. Although the members are appointed by Agency for Healthcare Research and Quality, USPSTF does not operate under FACA. The USPSTF Procedure Manual explicitly outlines how members' financial and nonfinancial conflicts of interest are identified and managed (USPSTF, 2015b). Briefly, potential conflicts are graded as levels 1, 2, or 3. The conflict's level corresponds to recommended actions regarding public disclosure of the conflict and the extent to which the member should participate in discussions and voting on the specific matter. The period of disclosure for conflicts is the 36 months prior to completing the form, which is in contrast to the previous 12 months asked for on OGE Form 450. All publications related to the topic under consideration must be disclosed, regardless of when they were published. The USPSTF website lists all conflicts classified as level 3, along with the action taken because of the disqualifying activity (USPSTF, 2015a).

European Food Safety Authority

The European Food Safety Authority (EFSA) is an independent agency funded by the European Union to serve as a source of scientific advice and communication on risks related to the food chain. The procedure for identifying and handling potential conflict of interests delineates how financial and scientific interests are managed, while a separate guidance document provides definitions and instructions on what needs to be declared (EFSA, 2009a,b). A general declaration of interests must be completed annually, while a specific declaration must be submitted before each meeting that is tailored to the specific topic to be discussed at that meeting. Members, the chair, hearing experts, and staff are all asked to submit declarations, which are all made available to the public.

EFSA notes that scientific expertise is necessary to fulfill its mission and tasks and that requisite experiences are understood to be part of being an expert; interests are therefore not necessarily considered a conflict of interest. The disclosure period is the 5 years prior to completing the declaration. The forms ask members to state (1) ownership or other investments, (2) member of a managing body or equivalent structure, (3) member of a scientific advisory body, (4) employment, (5) consultancy/advisory, (6) research funding, (7) intellectual property, (8) other membership or affiliation, and (9) interests of close family members (EFSA, 2009b). Interests are graded as levels A (nonexistent), B (possible), or C (existent). Level B conflicts are managed by limiting the person's involvement (e.g., respond to specific questions, but cannot actively participate in final decision making). Level C conflicts require the person to be excluded from the activity and be replaced by another expert, but in exceptional cases a waiver can be granted (EFSA, 2009a).

World Health Organization Global Advisory Committee on Vaccine Safety

The Global Advisory Committee on Vaccine Safety is a standing committee that advises the World Health Organization (WHO). Members serve as individuals and cannot be affiliated with industry (WHO, 2016). Before serving on the advisory committee, members must complete the "Declaration of interest for WHO experts" form (WHO, 2014). The form asks the member to report employment and consulting appointments (previous 4 years), research support (previous 4 years), investment interests (valued at more than $5,000), intellectual property, and public statements and positions (previous 3 years). The form notes that a conflict does not necessarily disqualify an individual from service. The WHO secretariat may apply one of the following three measures for members with potential or significant conflicts: (1) publicly disclose the conflict and allow the member to fully participate; (2) prohibit the member's participation in portions of the advisory committee's work related to the conflict; and (3) total exclusion from the advisory committee's work. Members are required to disclose significant conflicts to other participants in the activity. The advisory committee's reports and publications all publish disclosed conflicts and remedies.

Australian Government National Health and Medical Research Council

The National Health and Medical Research Council (NHMRC) is commissioned under Australian law to develop evidence-based guidelines in population health, ethics, and clinical practice, and carries out this task through appointing expert task-based committees (NHMRC, 2014a).[8] The NHMRC's process for vetting candidates includes (1) identifying and disclosing potential conflicts of interest, including financial, intellectual, and organizational; (2) determining whether a conflict of interest exists; and (3) putting procedures in place to manage any conflicts of interest (NHMRC, 2012). Financial activities to be reported include employment (previous 3 years), ownership interests (for the member and his or her immediate family), and consulting fees, honorarium, grants, travel support, meals and beverages, entertainment, gifts and gratuities, and any other financial interest (for the member and his or her immediate family; previous 3 years and anticipated in the 12 months that follow). Candidates are also asked to report relevant professional and organizational experience (e.g., publications, speeches or lectures, expert testimony, development of related guidelines and materials) and any other affiliations, relationships, or associations that could be perceived as a potential conflict. Conflicts are disclosed in writing to the chief executive officer or delegate, and they are disclosed verbally in a discussion with the membership, upon which the presiding individual determines appointment and appropriate management procedures if necessary. The NHMRC's chief executive officer is responsible for overseeing this process, but he or she has the authority to delegate this responsibility to a committee member or NHMRC staff member (NHMRC, 2012). The committee chair, who also must be free of conflicts of interest, is responsible for overseeing the compliance to any management plans. Committee member declarations of conflicts and any management plans put in place are published on the NHMRC website on an ongoing basis (conflict declarations are updated every meeting), unless an exception is granted by the chief executive officer, as well as published in the final guidelines (NHMRC, 2014b).

[8]National Health and Medical Research Council Act, Act No. 25, 1992, Australian government.

American College of Chest Physicians Antithrombotic Guidelines, Ninth Edition

Professional organizations also offer examples of differing selection processes, although not always in the context of an advisory committee. While many professional organizations put together advisory committees, not all have a strong record on conflicts of interest. Many professional organizations follow generally similar processes, including not hosting a public comment session and requiring committee members to be a member of the host organization. This National Academies committee identified one example notable for its unique process: the development of the ninth edition of antithrombotic guidelines, convened by the American College of Chest Physicians. Specifically, this professional organization explicitly reviews intellectual conflicts of interest. In composing this committee, the conveners developed management strategies to balance conflicts of interest with the expertise needed to develop the guidelines. Each committee member disclosed both financial and intellectual conflicts in writing for each recommendation, and the conflicts were reviewed and graded as either primary or secondary by the American College of Chest Physicians Health and Science Policy Committee. Primary conflicts, such as consultancies or authorship of original studies directly related to the recommendations in question, were considered serious and required management plans, including recusal from voting on recommendations (Guyatt et al., 2012). Secondary conflicts, such as consultancies not directly related to the recommendations in question, or participation in previous guidelines panels, were considered less serious and did not require a management plan. The Health and Science Policy Committee did not enforce the recusal of conflicted experts throughout its deliberations; this was managed by a nonconflicted methodologist who co-led each content area with a relevant, but generally conflicted, content expert (Guyatt et al., 2012). In this example, although conflicts were identified in the committee selection process, the Health and Science Policy Committee relied on the management plan in place to produce guidelines free of undue influence from conflicts of interest (Akl et al., 2014). Conflicts for each recommendation were published in the final guidelines.

CONCLUSION

This National Academies committee's review of selection processes revealed profound variation across several steps of selection processes, including membership types, methods for soliciting nominations, and the ways in which candidates are screened, vetted, and appointed. Among committees that are required to abide by FACA, practices were found to range widely by agency. Even less agreement was identified in the development of nonfederal advisory committees. Because this committee could not identify valid measures of success and a lack of standardization, no set of best practices were recognized. Instead, interesting examples were identified for promoting transparency, as well as for including a range of viewpoints and expertise in an advisory committee.

There are many methods to broaden committee membership and enhance transparency not used by the DGAC. For example, one approach is to use different types of committee member designations (i.e., special government employee, regular government employee, representative, ex officio, nonvoting members). Committees have enhanced their transparency through documentation and public release of information. Stages of the process where this has been accomplished includes the solicitation of nominations from the public and procedures for identifying and managing conflicts of interest. While the assessment of financial conflicts is standard, evaluating nonfinancial conflicts appears to pose a greater challenge. Some groups have created forms and questionnaires in an effort to capture and document these relatively subjective potential influences. The selection authority and process typically resides with the convening entity, although outside offices or organizations have been consulted in the appointment process.

REFERENCES

AHRQ (Agency for Healthcare Research and Quality). 2015. *AHRQ evidence-based practice center policy on financial and nonfinancial interests.* https://effectivehealthcare.ahrq.gov/about/epc (accessed October 5, 2017).

Akl, E. A., P. El-Hachem, H. Abou-Haidar, I. Neumann, H. J. Schunemann, and G. H. Guyatt. 2014. Considering intellectual, in addition to financial, conflicts of interest proved important in a clinical practice guideline: A descriptive study. *Journal of Clinical Epidemiology* 67(11):1222-1228.

Bero, L. 2014. What is in a name? Nonfinancial influences on the outcomes of systematic reviews and guidelines. *Journal of Clinical Epidemiology* 67(11):1239-1241.

Boyd, E. A., and L. A. Bero. 2006. Improving the use of research evidence in guideline development: 4. Managing conflicts of interests. *Health Research Policy and Systems* 4.

Boyd, E. A., E. A. Akl, M. Baumann, J. R. Curtis, M. J. Field, R. Jaeschke, M. Osborne, and H. J. Schunemann. 2012. Guideline funding and conflicts of interest: Article 4 in integrating and coordinating efforts in COPD guideline development. An official ATS/ERS workshop report. *Proceedings of the American Thoracic Society* 9(5):234-242.

CRS (Congressional Research Service). 2007. *Federal advisory committees: A primer.* https://fas.org/sgp/crs/misc/RL30260.pdf (accessed October 5, 2017).

DHS (U.S. Department of Homeland Security). 2011. Homeland Security Information Network Advisory Committee. *Federal Register* 76(212):67581-68055.

DOC (U.S. Department of Commerce). 2012. *Census Bureau National Advisory Committee on Racial, Ethnic, and Other Populations membership balance plan.* https://www.facadatabase.gov/rpt/_message.asp (accessed October 5, 2017).

DOC. 2015. *OGC FACA membership.* https://ogc.commerce.gov/page/faca-membership (accessed October 5, 2017).

DOC. 2016a. *Charter of the Census Bureau National Advisory Committee on Racial, Ethnic and Other Populations.* https://www.facadatabase.gov/rpt/_message.asp (accessed October 5, 2017).

DOC. 2016b. Request for nominations of members to serve on the National Advisory Committee on Racial, Ethnic, and Other Populations. *Federal Register* 81(115):39022-39023.

DOL (U.S. Department of Labor). 2015a. *Advisory Board on Toxic Substances and Worker Health charter.* https://www.dol.gov/owcp/energy/regs/compliance/AdvisoryBoard.htm (accessed October 5, 2017).

DOL. 2015b. Advisory Board on Toxic Substances and Worker Health notice of comment period. *Federal Register* 80(199):62111-62113.

DOL. 2015c. Advisory Board on Toxic Substances and Worker Health, notice of advisory board establishment. *Federal Register* 80(139):43292.

DOL. 2015d. *Membership balance plan.* Advisory Board on Toxic Substances and Worker Health to Part E of the Energy Employees Occupational Illness Compensation Program Act (EEOICPA). https://www.dol.gov/owcp/energy/regs/compliance/AdvisoryBoard.htm (accessed October 5, 2017).

EFSA (European Food Safety Authority). 2009a. *Implementing act to the policy on declaration of interests: Procedure for identifying and handling potential conflicts of interest.* http://www.efsa.europa.eu/sites/default/files/efsa_rep/blobserver_assets/doiconflicts.pdf (accessed January 3, 2017).

EFSA. 2009b. *Implementing act to the policy on declaration of interests: Guidance document on declarations of interest.* http://www.efsa.europa.eu/sites/default/files/efsa_rep/blobserver_assets/doiguidance.pdf (accessed January 3, 2017).

EPA (U.S. Environmental Protection Agency). 2015a. *Chemical Safety Advisory Committee charter.* https://www.epa.gov/tsca-peer-review/chemical-safety-advisory-committee-charter (accessed October 5, 2017).

EPA. 2015b. Chemical Safety Advisory Committee; establishment of a federal advisory committee; request for nominations. *Federal Register* 80(113):33517-33518.

EPA. 2015c. *Establishment of a federal advisory committee.* https://www.regulations.gov/docketBrowser?rpp=50&so=DESC&sb=postedDate&po=0&dct=PS&D=EPA-HQ-OPPT-2015-0233 (accessed October 5, 2017).

EPA. 2015d. *Membership balance plan.* Chemical Safety Advisory Committee. http://www.csg.org/aapca/documents/CSACMembershipBalancePlan2015.pdf (accessed October 5, 2017).

EPA. 2016. *Confidential financial disclosure form for Environmental Protection Agency special government employees (EPA form 3110-48).* https://www.epa.gov/sap/confidential-financial-disclosure-form-environmental-protection-agency-special-government (accessed October 5, 2017).

FDA (U.S. Food and Drug Administration). 2016. *FDA advisory committee membership application.* https://www.accessdata.fda.gov/scripts/FACTRSPortal/FACTRS/index.cfm (accessed October 5, 2017).

FDIC (Federal Deposit Insurance Corporation). 2014. *Charter of the FDIC Advisory Committee on Economic Inclusion.* https://www.fdic.gov/about/comein (accessed October 5, 2017).

GAO (U.S. Government Accountability Office). 2004. *Federal advisory committees: Additional guidance could help agencies better ensure independence and balance.* (GAO-04-328). Washington, DC: GAO Office of Public Affairs.

GAO. 2015. Physician-focused Payment Model Technical Advisory Committee nomination letters. *Federal Register* 80(110):32562.

GSA (U.S. General Services Administration). 2016. *FACA database.* http://www.facadatabase.gov (accessed October 5, 2017).

Guyatt, G., E. A. Akl, J. Hirsh, C. Kearon, M. Crowther, D. Gutterman, S. Z. Lewis, I. Nathanson, R. Jaeschke, and H. Schünemann. 2010. The vexing problem of guidelines and conflict of interest: A potential solution. *Annals of Internal Medicine* 152(11):738-741.

Guyatt, G. H., S. L. Norris, S. Schulman, J. Hirsh, M. H. Eckman, E. A. Akl, M. Crowther, P. O. Vandvik, J. W. Eikelboom, M. S. McDonagh, S. Z. Lewis, D. D. Gutterman, D. J. Cook, and H. J. Schünemann. 2012. Methodology for the development of antithrombotic therapy and prevention of thrombosis guidelines: Antithrombotic therapy and prevention of thrombosis, 9th ed. American College of Chest Physicians evidence-based clinical practice guidelines. *Chest* 141(2 Suppl):53S-70S.

HHS (U.S. Department of Health and Human Services). 2009. *Amended charter: HIT policy committee.* https://www.healthit.gov/hitac/health-it-policy-committee (accessed October 5, 2017).

HHS. 2014a. *FACA membership application.* https://www.healthit.gov/facas/faca-workgroup-membership-application (accessed October 5, 2017).

HHS. 2014b. Solicitation of nominations for membership on the National Vaccine Advisory Committee. *Federal Register* 79(82):23977-23979.

HHS. 2015a. *Charter of the 2015 Dietary Guidelines Advisory Committee.* https://health.gov/Dietaryguidelines/dgac2015-charter-final.pdf (accessed October 5, 2017).

HHS. 2015b. *Charter of the Healthcare Infection Control Practices Advisory Committee.* https://www.cdc.gov/hicpac/charter.html (accessed October 5, 2017).

HHS. 2015c. Health IT Policy Committee and Health IT Standards Committee; call for applications. *Federal Register* 80(153):47935-47936.

HHS. 2015d. *Membership balance plan.* Healthcare Infection Control Practices Advisory Committee (HICPAC). https://www.cdc.gov/hicpac/about.html (accessed October 5, 2017).

HHS. 2015e. *National Vaccine Advisory Committee charter.* https://www.hhs.gov/nvpo/nvac/charter/index.html (accessed October 5, 2017).

HHS. 2015f. *Membership balance plan.* National Vaccine Advisory Committee. https://www.hhs.gov/nvpo/nvac/charter/index.html (accessed October 5, 2017).

HHS. 2015g. Request for nomination for industry representatives and participation from industry organizations on public advisory committees. *Federal Register* 80(72):20233-20235.

HHS. 2016a. *Arthritis Advisory Committee charter.* https://www.fda.gov/AdvisoryCommittees/CommitteesMeetingMaterials/Drugs/ArthritisAdvisoryCommittee/ucm094137.htm (accessed October 5, 2017).

HHS. 2016b. *Membership balance plan.* Arthritis Advisory Committee. https://www.fda.gov/AdvisoryCommittees/CommitteesMeetingMaterials/Drugs/ArthritisAdvisoryCommittee/ucm094137.htm (accessed October 5, 2017).

HHS. 2016c. *Physician-focused payment model technical advisory Committee: Bylaws.* https://aspe.hhs.gov/physician-focused-payment-model-technical-advisory-committee-bylaws (accessed October 5, 2017).

HHS. 2016d. Request for nominations of candidates to serve on the Healthcare Infection Control Practices Advisory Committee (HICPAC). *Federal Register* 81(86):26797-26798.

HHS/USDA (U.S. Department of Agriculture). 2012. Announcement of the intent to establish the 2015 Dietary Guidelines Advisory Committee and solicitation of nominations for appointment to the Committee membership. *Federal Register* 77(208):65384-65385.

IOM (Institute of Medicine). 2009. *Conflict of interest in medical research, education, and practice.* Washington, DC: The National Academies Press.

Jacobson, P. 2016 (unpublished). *Approaches to bias and conflict of interest-how would you suggest minimizing conflicts of interest and "eliminating bias" while preserving a wide range of viewpoints.* Presentation to the Committee to Review the Process to Update the *Dietary Guidelines for Americans*.

NASS (USDA National Agriculture Statistics Service). 2016. Solicitation of nominations to the advisory Committee on agriculture statistics. *Federal Register* 81(210):75372-75373.

NHMRC (National Health and Medical Research Council). 2012. *Guideline development and conflicts of interest: Identifying and managing conflicts of interest of prospective members and members of NHMRC committees and working groups developing guidelines.* Commonwealth of Australia: National Health and Medical Research Council. https://www.nhmrc.gov.au/guidelines-publications/information-guideline-developers/guideline-development-and-conflicts-interes (accessed October 5, 2017).

NHMRC. 2014a. *How NHMRC develops its guidelines.* Australian government. https://www.nhmrc.gov.au/guidelines-publications/how-nhmrc-develops-its-guidelines (accessed October 5, 2017).

NHMRC. 2014b. *NHMRC form for disclosure of interests (guideline development).* Australian government. https://www.nhmrc.gov.au/_files_nhmrc/file/guidelines/developers/doi_interactive_guideline_development_140331.pdf (accessed October 5, 2017).

OGE (U.S. Office of Government Ethics). 2000. *Summary of ethical requirements applicable to special government employees.* https://www2.oge.gov/Web/OGE.nsf/Resources/DO-00-003:+Summary+of+Ethical+Requirements+Applicable+to+Special+Government+Employees (accessed October 5, 2017).

OGE. 2015. *OGE Form 450: Confidential financial disclosure report.* https://oge.gov/Web/oge.nsf/Resources/OGE+Form+450:+Confidential+Financial+Disclosure+Report (accessed October 5, 2017).

USDA (U.S. Department of Agriculture). 2016a. *Advisory Committee on Agriculture Statistics charter.* https://www.federalregister.gov/documents/2016/08/31/2016-20899/advisory-committee-on-agriculture-statistics (accessed October 5, 2017).

USDA. 2016b. *Membership balance plan.* Advisory Committee on Agriculture Statistics. https://www.federalregister.gov/documents/2016/08/31/2016-20899/advisory-committee-on-agriculture-statistics (accessed October 5, 2017).

USDA/HHS. 2016 (unpublished). Dietary Guidelines for Americans: *Process brief, sections 1–3.* Prepared for the Committee to Review the Process to Update the *Dietary Guidelines for Americans.*

USPSTF (U.S. Preventive Services Task Force). 2015a. *Conflict of interest disclosures.* https://www.uspreventiveservicestaskforce.org/Page/Name/conflict-of-interest-disclosures (accessed October 5, 2017).

USPSTF. 2015b. *U.S. Preventive Services Task Force procedure manual.* https://www.uspreventiveservicestaskforce.org/Home/GetFile/6/7/procedure-manual_2015/pdf (accessed October 5, 2017).

WHO (World Health Organization). 2014. *Declaration of interests for WHO experts form.* http://www.who.int/about/declaration-of-interests/en (accessed October 5, 2017).

WHO. 2016. *Global Advisory Committee on Vaccine Safety terms of reference.* http://www.who.int/vaccine_safety/committee/en (accessed October 5, 2017).

4

Opportunities to Build Trust

It is not uncommon for guidance related to controversial issues to be questioned, especially when many stakeholders are involved. In such cases, the steps for how the guidance was developed are just as important to support the integrity of the process as the guidance itself. On the whole, this National Academies of Sciences, Engineering, and Medicine (the National Academies) committee believes the current selection process—identifying individuals and creating a diverse panel—can reasonably lead to the appointment of a fair and balanced Dietary Guidelines Advisory Committee (DGAC). However, this National Academies committee believes the selection process for DGAC members needs to be enhanced to optimize its integrity.

ASSESSMENT OF THE DGAC SELECTION PROCESS

The evidentiary base is limited for identifying characteristics of selection processes that most effectively address key concerns, such as diversity and balance. As such, to conduct an independent review of the DGAC selection process, this National Academies committee relied on assessments of good practices from other organizations (see Chapter 3) and its own collective expertise and experience. From an assessment of these sources emerged a set of values the committee believes could enhance the integrity of a selection process:

- *Enhance transparency.* The foremost important characteristic of an effective process for the selection of advisory committee members is transparency. To the extent practicable, each step ought to be described in as much detail as possible and be made available to the public for its understanding. This transparency can help reassure the public that no undue influences or untoward actions are being taken.
- *Promote diversity of expertise and experience.* A broad range of expertise and experience must be considered to create a balanced committee. Expertise has to align with the topic areas to be reviewed. Diversity with respect to nontechnical skills (e.g., ability to form consensus or develop compromise) also needs to be considered. Building on the first characteristic of transparency, involvement from a broad range of perspectives, including public involvement, is also critical to fostering diversity.
- *Support a deliberative process.* A deliberative process should be used that considers information from a wide variety of sources. Decision makers ought to freely exchange information with one another toward the goal of coming to agreement or consensus. To the extent possible, the public should be engaged as well.
- *Manage biases and conflicts of interest.* The biases of individual members should be balanced among a broad representation of perspectives. Actual and or perceived conflicts of interest—both financial and nonfinancial—should be eliminated to the extent possible or their effects be minimized.
- *Adopt state-of-the-art processes and methods.* As practicable, selection processes and actions ought to be based on the best available evidence for the broader purpose of managing bias and conflict of interest. They should be revised and improved on as new evidence arises.

This National Academies committee used these five values of an "ideal" selection process to assess the current DGAC selection process. The discussions in the following sections describe that assessment, recognizing that each characteristic does not necessarily apply to every step of the process.

Overall, this National Academies committee found that the DGAC selection process is a thoughtful process that works within the bounds of the relevant laws to serve the U.S. Department of Agriculture (USDA) and the U.S. Department of Health and Human Services (HHS), as well as the American public. However, as noted in Chapter 1, the lack of transparency in the current process could lead to the perception that the membership of the DGAC is inequitable, which affects its integrity and trustworthiness.

Perception can be just as important as the truth when earning the public's trust. How the process is perceived cannot be controlled, but the process can be engineered to show that it is thoughtful, fair, and supports the task. The selection process has been focused on appointing a group of experts able to assess the evidence related to nutrition and health. Based on critiques of previous DGACs and the significant nature of their work, this National Academies committee believes a shift may be warranted such that the selection process also focuses on engendering trust from the public. These proposed additions to the existing process would address the perception that the selection process is currently "obscure and not transparent" (Willett, 2016).

The current DGAC selection process consists of nine steps beginning with the establishment of a charter and culminating in the swearing in of the members (see Figure 2-1). This National Academies committee's assessment of the process focused on step 3: Conduct a review of nominations and propose a slate of candidates. The other steps reasonably meet the goals delineated by the committee.

The processes used to establish the charter follow the guidelines laid out to support implementation of the Federal Advisory Committee Act (FACA), such as publishing a notice in the *Federal Register*. The nominations process also involves receipt of input from a broad range of stakeholders, including the public, allowing candidates to be identified with various expertise and experience. The call for nominations is sent to various online mailing lists, but ought to be shared even more broadly throughout the nutrition and health policy communities, for example through publication in relevant journals and social media, to broaden the pool of candidates. There are relatively few drawbacks to expanding the call for nominations, especially when using fast and inexpensive technologies, but would have the probable advantages of improving diversity of expertise and experience.

The third step—conduct a review of nominations and propose a slate of candidates—is not as transparent as it could be, and not much information is publicly available about the basis for the selections that are made. Many of the processes used to complete these steps are currently described publicly at a high level. For example, the membership balance plan for the 2015 DGAC states that its members would be balanced across many dimensions, including diversity across geographic areas, academic institutions, gender, race, ethnicity, and disability. However, this National Academies committee's review of previous DGACs found a preponderance of DGAC members from the northeast, while noting inclusion of several members from the midwest and south. However, geographic diversity will likely be an ongoing issue.

As this third step is perhaps the most subjective step in the selection process, and is arguably the most critical, it ought to be made even clearer to the public. Discussions about how individual nominees were considered with respect to their qualifications against selection criteria could be disclosed to the public. How perspectives on the advisory committee are balanced could be shared publicly. The membership balance plan outlines the process and criteria against which candidates are screened for selection, but the high-level descriptions in the plan could provide more detail to foster trust and integrity in the process. Also unclear is how closely the membership balance plan is followed in the development of the DGAC and how well the plan is implemented.

Specific to consideration of biases and conflicts of interest, how USDA and HHS approach these concepts is not clear. A review of conflicts of interest is mentioned as part of the process for special government employees, but more specific information could describe how conflicts of interest are identified in selection of the DGAC and, if needed, how they will be managed. Understanding how biases and conflicts of interest are identified and managed through a deliberative process would provide more transparency to the public on vetting and selecting advisory committee members. This National Academies committee identified this third step as an opportunity to enhance transparency and inclusiveness, as well as minimize undue influences (see Figure 4-1). The remainder of this chapter lays out this committee's suggestions and specific recommendations for modifying the DGAC selection process.

ENHANCE TRANSPARENCY DURING CANDIDATE REVIEW

"Conduct a review of nominations and propose a slate of candidates" (see step 3 in Figure 2-1) is inherently the most subjective step in the current DGAC selection process. The perception by some is that the entire selection process is influenced by political interests since the secretaries from both USDA and HHS are political appointments, and the fact that USDA also supports U.S. agriculture (Mozaffarian, 2016). However, this National Academies committee was unable to identify any hard evidence that the *Dietary Guidelines for Americans* (*DGA*) have been unduly influenced because of USDA's potential conflict. Unfortunately, there are limited objective measures to judge a nominee's qualifications and the overall balance of a committee. In such subjective matters, the public must trust in the veracity of the process to achieve dependable results. Full transparency in the form of publicly accessible deliberations about every nominee is not practical given the sensitivity around why someone is or is not considered a strong candidate for DGAC membership. For example, considerations of personal finances, past history and relationships, and personal beliefs are all included in these deliberations. In part

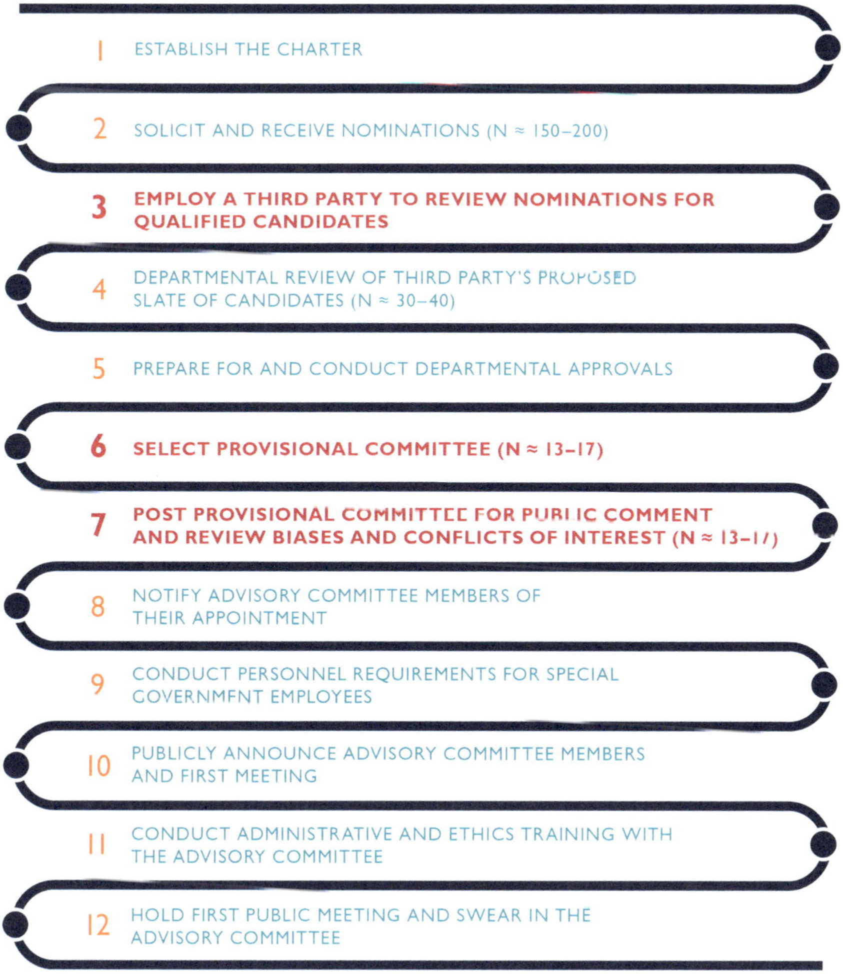

FIGURE 4-1 Proposed process for selecting the Dietary Guidelines Advisory Committee.
NOTE: Steps highlighted in red are new, proposed steps.
SOURCE: Abstracted from USDA/HHS, 2016a.

because of these constraints, there may be the perception that the departments are not fairly considering all qualified candidates and not including representation of a broad spectrum of perspectives (Gummalla, 2016; Maitin-Shepard, 2016). This National Academies committee deliberated three options for improving the openness of this step.

Candidate Review Option 1

The first option this National Academies committee considered was to continue the status quo, where USDA and HHS vet nominees and appoint members. However, options for how to improve the current selection process, while keeping the full process under USDA and HHS, would likely result in marginal improvements. A different tactic would be needed to resolve the questions raised about the equity and integrity of the selection and appointment of members in a meaningful way. This option would be budget neutral and would likely continue to result in a 6- to 7-month process.

Candidate Review Option 2

One way to reduce the bias and perceived influence of political interests in the DGAC is to remove the selection process entirely from USDA and HHS. This would involve finding a third party that could identify and review all candidates and develop and appoint a balanced panel of experts. This approach is taken by HHS for its Physician-Focused Payment Model Technical Advisory Committee, where, by statute, the Comptroller General of the United States appoints members (HHS, 2016).[1] Of note, FACA requires that unless called for by statute, presidential directive, or other establishment authority, the final authority to select members rests with the agency heads, which in this case is the secretaries.[2] Changing the appointment authority for the DGAC would either require legislative action or a presidential directive.

The third party would need to be an objective arbiter with a strong record of having both the theoretical knowledge and practical expertise of having assembled impartial, neutral committees. It could be a private, nonprofit, or government organization, but it should not be part of either of the sponsoring agencies. In this option, a third party would also need to have expertise in the areas affected by the *DGA* in order to properly balance perspectives.

---

[1]The U.S. Government Accountability Office serves in this role for a number of committees, but these are the only federal advisory committees to which it makes appointments (personal communication, M. Giffin, U.S. Government Accountability Office, September 21, 2016). The Medicaid and Children's Health Insurance Program Payment and Access Commission, Medicare Payment Advisory Committee, Patient-Centered Outcomes Research Institute Governing Board, Patient-Centered Outcomes Research Institute Methodology Committee, and Physician-Focused Payment Model Technical Advisory Committee memberships are all appointed by the Comptroller General of the United States (GAO, 2016). Appointments to the Health Information Technology Policy Committee are also made by congressional leaders.

[2]Federal Advisory Committee Act of 1972, 41 C.F.R. § 102-3.130(a).

There is no assurance that another body would not be subject to outside influences, while also being close enough to the subject matter to appropriately balance perspectives and expertise. This option would potentially require additional resources and would likely add months to the already tight time frame for selecting members.

Candidate Review Option 3

Another option would be to have the review and final selection be separated into two steps, conducted by two different bodies. A third party could be tasked with ensuring that a wide range of viewpoints and expertise was considered for the panel and objectively narrow down the list of nominees. Specifically, it could consider candidates' nomination packages and qualifications, identify other candidates as necessary, interview promising candidates, provide an initial cursory review of biases and conflicts of interest, and submit a slate of primary and alternate nominees for the secretaries' consideration. With its experience in the field, USDA and HHS could still be responsible for the role of balancing expertise and perspectives for final selection. The departments could provide the third party with selection criteria for nominees to maintain continuity in the process. These criteria ought to be shared publicly as part of the description of balance to be filed in accordance with FACA.

Although it is uncommon for other organizations to conduct all the steps and not be the final appointing authority for a federal advisory committee, the National Vaccine Advisory Committee may provide a model for a more limited third party role in committee selection. In this case, the legislation states that the National Academy of Sciences (NAS) will review the small number of nominees received for each vacancy (HHS, 2015). Candidates' subject-matter expertise are considered during this assessment, but a review of potential conflicts of interest resides with the federal government. It is anticipated that once a third party is identified and employed, the review process would take up to 4 months to complete. Additional time would be required for the departmental selections and approval processes.

A third party, as discussed in option 2, would need to be an organization without a political, economic, or ideological identity. Preferably, the organization would have a history of putting together well-respected, impartial panels of experts. Unlike option 2, since the third party would not be making final selections, it would not necessarily need to be expert in nutrition or dietary guidance, just expert in evaluating individuals' expertise and experience. This would allow for a wider range of possible third-party organizations to be considered.

Many types of organizations could possibly serve as a third party for narrowing down the candidate pool, including other government agencies, consulting companies, nonpartisan research and policy groups, or professional organizations. Options within the government ought to include agencies outside of the sponsoring departments, such as agencies of Congress. Private-sector options include nonprofit, not-for-profit, and for-profit organizations. Regardless of what type of organization is chosen, an examination of a private-sector organization's funding sources and customer bases would help ensure impartiality. A third party would need to consider a wide variety of members, not just members of potential host organizations, a common practice identified for professional organizations, as discussed in Chapter 3. A thorough search for an appropriate external organization would be required.

There are advantages of using an unbiased third party with the characteristics delineated above. This National Academies committee's opinion is that political bias—both the perception and reality—would be reduced by a third party since USDA and HHS would not be involved in narrowing the field of candidates. If the secretaries of USDA and HHS are selecting final nominees from a short list of equally well-qualified, nonconflicted candidates, there is a greater potential that the final DGAC will be neutral. This in fact has the potential to reduce bias but even stronger potential to improve perception. Having the secretaries continue to select the final membership would also remove the need for the external organization to have expertise related to the *DGA*, likely resulting in a broader pool of candidates.

This alternative also has drawbacks like those delineated in option 2. There is no absolute guarantee that a third party will reduce bias; there is no evidence to say that a third party would not come up with the same exact committee of experts as assembled by the current process. Additionally, the secretaries of USDA and HHS remain the appointing authorities under this option. However, to the many critics of the process, a third party would ensure that USDA and HHS were more at an arm's length from the selection of DGAC members. This committee believes that at the very least, this would improve public perception of a more objective process, as the mandate from Congress indicates that some subsets of the public do not trust the *DGA*. Another drawback is that this option would also likely have budgetary implications despite some savings in staff time, as well as lengthen the selection process. However, selection of a third party could begin before the charter is filed so as to leave the DGAC with as much time as possible to conduct its work.

Conclusion

This National Academies committee recognizes few objective measures exist to assess the effectiveness of a selection process. In considering the options, the committee could not find explicit evidence to suggest that the current process is biased, but also accepts that there is no explicit evidence to prove that it is not. Continuing the status quo would result in an unsatisfactory response to the fundamental issue of how the full list of nominees is narrowed down to the final committee and does not suggest option 1 be selected. The committee concludes that the current process needs to be more transparent than it currently is to assure the public that a wide set of viewpoints and expertise is being considered. However, the committee does not believe that the appointment authority needs to be removed from the secretaries of USDA and HHS, and therefore does not believe option 2 is the best approach.

This National Academies committee envisions that a hybrid approach be adopted as outlined in option 3 where a neutral, unbiased arbiter would be used as a first screen, still leaving responsibility for balancing the final advisory committee and appointing members with the secretaries. At a minimum, this National Academies committee believes divorcing the screening process from the appointment authority would improve perception that the DGAC process is more neutral than it currently is. The committee believes the proposed separation of the processes also has the potential to actually reduce bias. This separation would be feasible immediately, as only a change to the appointing authority would require action from Congress or the president. Given the lack of available evidence, it is this National Academies committee's best judgment and opinion that the potential advantage of reducing bias and improving public perception would yield substantial benefits and believes the additional costs and time are important investments to make. No matter what option is chosen, the charter should be filed at the latest possible point to allow the DGAC as much time as possible to develop its report.

Recommendation 1. The secretaries of USDA and HHS should employ an external third party to review and narrow the candidate pool to a list of primary and alternate nominees. Criteria against which nominees are screened should be developed by USDA and HHS for use by the third party.

CRITERIA FOR SELECTING CANDIDATES

The criteria against which candidates are reviewed are discussed in this section. How composition is balanced and how expertise is considered are addressed in the next section. In the current process, candidates are assessed "based upon their qualifications, level of expertise and knowledge, and ability to contribute to the work to be performed," as well as diversity of "geographic areas, academic institutions, gender, race, ethnicity, and disability" (USDA/HHS, 2016a). Other factors are likely considered during the balancing process, but are not explicitly stated. Conflicts of interest and background checks are considered prior to appointment to the advisory committee.

Other factors are likely considered during the balancing process, but they are not explicitly stated. Additional criteria for considering candidates ought to include willingness to serve; minimal financial and nonfinancial conflicts of interest (see Boxes 3-2 and 3-3); biases that can be balanced with those of other members; and prior experience working on advisory committees or panels. Conflicts of interest and biases will be discussed in greater detail later in the chapter. Prior experience on panels is one important factor to evaluate the candidate's interpersonal skills. A binary yes or no account of past service on a committee is often the only measure of past committee experience, but the quality of that participation is more difficult to assess and measure. The committee intends for this criterion to include an assessment of interpersonal skills such as ability to compromise and collaborate, and ability to express and reconcile divergent opinions. Such skills can best be gauged by seeking feedback regarding the candidate's performance on prior consensus-developing activities. USDA and HHS could consider making all criteria available for public comment before adoption, if time allows. Receiving feedback on selection criteria could improve transparency, but would add more time to an already lengthy process to set up the advisory committee, and therefore would leave the DGAC with less time to complete its work.

Currently, information regarding candidates' technical expertise is collected during the initial solicitation and consists of a statement of qualifications and a curriculum vitae or resume limited to 10 pages. The committee believes more directed information ought to be sought during the call for nominations for consideration during selection. This could include experience on relevant boards or panels, activities related to nutrition policy, consulting, appointment as chair or cochair of committees and study groups, elected positions, and relevant publications or presentations. One example for the types of information to include is the biosketch requested by the National Institutes of Health, which requests submission of a brief personal statement describing the candidate's qualifications for the particular project; list of positions and honors; statement of the candidate's most significant contributions to science; and additional information, such as research support and/or scholastic performance. The total length is limited to five pages (NIH, 2016).

The proposed chair, co-chairs, or vice chair would ideally be held to a higher standard as the leadership of the advisory committee and would not necessarily need to be a subject-matter expert (IOM, 2011). Although difficult to achieve, to the extent possible, it would be preferable if these individuals were not biased in the specific areas being addressed. Most importantly, these members need to be free of financial conflicts of interest, and nonfinancial conflicts of interest if possible. The proposed chair would also preferably have served in a leadership role for other panels or committees.

Currently, as the advisory committee's leader, the chair presides over meetings and serves as the liaison to the departments to help establish priorities. The chair also has a number of administrative duties, such as certifying accuracy of meeting minutes and requesting motions to vote. One important part of the role is to facilitate discussions. However, this can be difficult to do while also keeping focused on the substance of the deliberations. A facilitator could be used to guide the flow of discussions to ensure all members are heard. An effective facilitator would remain neutral, understand group dynamics, be flexible yet firm, know when to let the advisory committee work through an issue, and be sensitive to the politics at hand. Adding a facilitator would not be budget neutral, but could help the advisory committee complete its tasks in a more efficient manner. If a facilitator is used, facilitation skills would not need to be part of the criteria for selecting a chair. Otherwise, ability to facilitate a group ought to be a key criterion for choosing the leadership of the DGAC.

Skills need to be reviewed for the group as a whole, as well as individuals. The organization selecting candidates will need to review the collective expertise, experience, and perspectives before making final appointments. Through this deliberative process, the public can be assured that the advisory committee is objective and has the requisite expertise to complete its task.

DGAC COMPOSITION

As described in Chapter 2, in accordance with FACA, agencies are required to consider candidates from all backgrounds who are "directly affected, interested, and qualified, as appropriate to the nature and functions of the advisory committee." Advisory committees providing technical guidance should also include people with "demonstrated professional or personal qualifications and experience relevant to the functions and tasks to be performed."[3] The 2015 DGAC membership balance plan identifies a set of 17 specialty areas to be represented, ranging from osteoporosis to nutrition-related systematic review methodology. However,

[3]Federal Advisory Committee Act of 1972, 41 C.F.R. § 102-3.60(b)(3).

the charter states that the final advisory committee is not limited to the categories listed in the balance plan. The membership balance plan does not anticipate how that distribution will be achieved across or within specialty categories. It calls for experts to have experience in one or more of the areas, so a one-to-one match is not needed between category of expertise and DGAC members. The plan also states that individuals for the 2015 DGAC are selected to represent viewpoints of the scientific evidence, not of any specific stakeholder groups.

After discussing various approaches, this National Academies committee concludes that the DGAC should represent a wide variety of perspectives so that any group of experts with a similar composition could be appointed and derive the same findings. During this deliberation, the complicated question arose of which should be developed first: the specific questions to be answered by the DGAC or the areas of expertise needed to address the charge? These are interdependent steps, but one must come before the other. The current process relies on the DGAC to develop priority topics for review rather than for an a priori process to identify which updates and reviews are most critically needed, thus influencing the expertise needed on the DGAC. This National Academies committee discussed the potential value of focusing on specific topic areas that need revision or updating in the *DGA*. This situation would allow for concentration of expertise in key priority topics rather than all the expertise needed for review of the *complete DGA*. This issue was discussed and debated because of the need to focus on recommendations for pregnant women and children from birth to 24 months in the 2020–2025 edition of the *DGA*. However, to meet the short timeline for this first report, this National Academies committee was not able to formulate a specific recommendation on this approach or more broadly about the advisory committee's overall composition. The committee will address these issues in its second report when it can fully examine the charge to the DGAC and the overall *DGA* process.

The options below were discussed as potential strategies to address the 2020 DGAC composition, recognizing the limitations on the size of the advisory committee. Customarily, 13 to 17 members are appointed to the DGAC. Adding additional members may be able to help expand the number of viewpoints represented, but it might make it difficult to derive consensus and might potentially delay the delivery of the DGAC's final report. Thus, it appears there are more areas of expertise that could help inform the DGAC than can reasonably be managed on an advisory committee. It may be worth taking a different approach to identifying members that allows for consideration of a greater mix of individuals with both particular expertise in focused areas of nutrition, as well as including broad, more general thinkers. Inclusion of other types of federal advisory committee members (e.g., representative members, nonvoting members; see Box 2-2) could also be considered as a way to improve buy-in and expand committee membership as needed. If these types of members are included in future DGACs, it would be critical to balance their areas of expertise and have a wide range of viewpoints included. USDA and HHS could consider improving transparency by publishing the categories of expertise each member represents.

Other perspectives could be included through use of non-DGAC member subcommittees, consultants, and invited speakers. In each of these situations, the invited experts would not have a voting role on the DGAC. Instead, their roles would be limited to helping inform the DGAC's deliberations and conclusions. Subcommittees could comprise outside experts and one or two DGAC members to make recommendations to the DGAC—not USDA or HHS—on broad questions requiring a number of areas of expertise. These subcommittees could be chaired by the one or two members of the DGAC. For more narrow topics not requiring a full subcommittee, or where the DGAC would like to supplement its expertise, consultants could be used. Because these individuals can influence decision making through the information provided to the DGAC for its deliberations, it is important that these participants provide balanced perspectives and that their conflicts of interest and biases are appropriately balanced and managed. The values identified by this National Academies committee to optimize the integrity of the process are important to consider for input from these non-DGAC members as well.

Multiple models for developing consensus were also discussed. For example, panels could consist of individuals knowledgeable in the topic area generally but not vested in the topic (e.g., through research or publicly stated opinions). Alternatively, it could comprise individuals with specialized expertise who are vested in and have published on the topic. New perspectives also could be considered, such as information management and systems science. These other disciplines can help bring innovations to the selection process. For example, an expert in new methods to manage information could bring about changes to the way candidates are reviewed, potentially minimizing the likelihood of bias and shortening the process for review. Another example includes modeling and simulation that could also be used to understand the potential long-term impacts of interventions that would not be possible to measure in the short-term.

ADDITIONAL PUBLIC COMMENT PERIODS

As discussed in Chapter 2, the current selection process seeks public comment through a call for nominations in the *Federal Register* and relevant online mailing lists (USDA/HHS, 2016a). Nominations are received from stakeholder groups from varying viewpoints. This National Academies committee concludes that this portion of the nomination process is strong and encourages transparency. However, the only formal opportunity for public input during the selection process is in response to the call for nominations. Another public comment period, targeted at nominees being considered for appointment, would improve the transparency of the DGAC selection process. Two models were considered for receiving additional public comments based on a review of other processes.

Public Comment Period Option 1

In addition to a public call for nomination, some agencies request public comments on qualified candidates. In this model, individuals identified during the nomination period would be posted on a website and/or the *Federal Register*. The public would be invited to comment on the candidates in terms of the overall balance of the advisory committee with respect to expertise and management of bias. All feedback would be taken into consideration during final selections, in addition to other relevant information either submitted during the nomination process (e.g., statements of qualifications, curriculum vitaes) or collected by staff. Based on the totality of information available, the appointing authority would select a panel of members.

This model is used to assemble some federal advisory committees, among others. For example, the U.S. Environmental Protection Agency (EPA) and the U.S. Department of Labor (DOL) have both invited the public to submit comments on lists of candidates.

EPA posted candidates' biographies for a 23-day comment period on the 72 nominees received for the Chemical Assessment Advisory Committee Augmented for Benzo[a]pyrene Review. Input received during that time was taken into consideration by the science advisory board's staff office director (EPA, 2014). The DOL Advisory Board on Toxic Substances and Worker Health holds a 14-day period when the public can submit comments to the secretary of labor about the qualifications of 66 nominees (DOL, 2015).

One benefit of this approach is that the full list of candidates would be disclosed to the public, allowing input to be received on any nominee. Decisions made by the appointing authority would be informed by evidence from all sources, whether brought forth by the individuals themselves, staff, or the public. While this enhances transparency in one regard, it still leaves in question considerations about how balance is achieved on the panel. Insights into how balance was achieved would only be made available to the public upon announcement of the full committee.

Public Comment Period Option 2

Another model this National Academies committee discussed was requesting input on a slate of provisional members. All necessary steps to finalize panel membership would be completed, but the appointment would be contingent upon consideration of public comments. Feedback would be invited for a reasonable period of time on the advisory committee's proposed composition. Appointments would not be finalized until after public comments were received and considered by the appointing authority. If comments indicated a provisional member had an intractable conflict or revealed previously unknown biases that could not be balanced, the department could confer with the provisional member, and if needed, reconsider the appointment. An approach like this is mandated by Section 15 of FACA for committees appointed by the NAS and the National Academy of Public Administration as described in Chapter 3. If identification of another member was warranted, an alternate member identified in prior steps could be selected and subjected to the same process as other provisional members. A separate public comment period could be held to provide opportunity to review the entire revised committee's composition. Use of multiple public comment periods would help minimize scrutiny as to why one person was originally listed as an alternate if the alternates are never turned to. It also reduces the burden on DGAC alternates by eliminating the need for these individuals to provide their entire history of potential conflicts of interest and reduces the possibility of unwarranted attacks.

This option promotes more complete public input than the current selection process by inviting feedback from all stakeholders on how the slate is balanced, as well as on potential individual members of the slate. Comments are encouraged to focus on both provisional members and the proposed committee as a whole. However, unlike the model discussed in option 1, the full list of candidates is not publicized; the public has to have confidence that provisional members were selected fairly.

Conclusion

Providing a reasonable amount of time for feedback is critical to a transparent process and the public should have an additional opportunity to comment after the initial solicitation of nominations (see step 7 of Figure 4-1). However, because allotting time for a public comment period does delay final appointments, the committee did not consider adding more than one opportunity for input.

This National Academies committee discussed the efficacy of the two options in the context of the DGAC. Over each of the past three cycles, the departments considered between 150 and 200 candidates (USDA/HHS, 2016b). In the past, the DGAC's lack of balance was criticized, and not necessarily for the qualifications of specific individuals (Maitin-Shepard, 2016). Considering the size of the candidate pool and the need to focus on the overall composition, the committee concluded that option 2 would more effectively address concerns raised by the public and encourage transparency.

Recommendation 2. The secretaries of USDA and HHS should make a list of provisional appointees open for public comment—including short biographies and any known conflicts—for a reasonable period of time prior to appointment.

All public comments about specific provisional members ought to be considered carefully. It is very likely that proposed membership would change as a result of the public comments and that a provisional member could be removed from or added to the slate. For the purpose of improving transparency, this National Academies committee did discuss posting public comments about each candidate, as well as explanations by USDA and HHS regarding why each primary and/or alternate candidate was or was not selected to serve on the DGAC. Candid information from the public about proposed members is critical for a deliberative process. However, posting such information would likely deter volunteers from wanting to serve on the DGAC. Although it is an honor to serve on such a prominent group, these individuals ultimately volunteer their time and expertise at their own will. Ad hominem attacks presented in public comments or in explanations by USDA or HHS could result in candidates being maligned in the public press and their reputations damaged, reducing the pool of qualified candidates willing to take part in such an activity. If USDA and HHS decide to share public comments made about each candidate, guidelines would need to be developed to protect candidates so that comments that are slanderous in nature would not be accepted for fear that they may be released, for example through a Freedom of Information Act request. In its review of other committee selection processes, this National Academies committee could not identify examples that make such information about candidates publicly available, and thus determined that the potential benefits were not substantial enough to warrant publication of all comments made about proposed members.

ADDRESSING BIASES AND CONFLICTS OF INTEREST

As discussed in Chapter 3, balancing biases and limiting conflicts of interest are both critical to establishing trust. This is particularly true in nutrition research, where industry, political influences, and professional organizations are all seen to be major sources of perceived conflict. Due to the lack of high-quality prospective cohort studies that directly impact the *DGA*, it would be difficult to eliminate these influences.

A policy explicitly stating how an organization will identify and manage conflicts is a standard tool used to combat perceptions of undue influence. In medicine, these policies aim "to protect the integrity of professional judgment and to preserve public trust rather than to try to remediate problems with bias or mistrust after they occur" (IOM, 2009, p. 28). Organizations around the world—including the federal government, medical journals, and universities—have adopted policies concerning conflicts of interest (Boyd et al., 2004; Graham et al., 2015).[4]

The literature review described in Chapter 1 on conflict of interest examined these specifically in relation to guideline development and advisory committees. Significant variation was observed across advisory committees and guideline development groups in how information on conflicts of interest was defined, collected, and managed. The literature broadly supports the notion that disclosure and management of conflicts of interest is a necessary part of establishing public trust and increasing transparency in guideline development (Barrow and Conrad, 2006; Gessner et al., 2010; Rowe et al., 2009, 2013; Schünemann et al., 2006, 2015). However, policies for disclosure and management vary across groups.

Financial disclosures are not widely published in guidelines (Bindslev et al., 2013; Khalil et al., 2012; Tibau et al., 2015) despite broad agreement that disclosure is beneficial in reducing the risk of and appearance of bias resulting from conflicts of interest (Rowe et al., 2009). Across organizations that have already implemented disclosure practices, examples of disclosure methods identified include verbal, written on a detailed form, and written in response to broad questions. Examples of groups to whom disclosure was reported include a third-party reviewer or oversight committee, others in the guideline development group, and/or public disclosure.

The evidence base directly linking disclosed conflicts of interest to associated outcomes is limited, in part, because of a lack of standardization on outcomes to assess. Potential outcomes can be framed as both positive and negative. Positive outcomes could be some measure of trustworthiness, reduced bias, or actual health outcomes. Negative outcomes could be lower-quality recommendations as a result of not including experts or missed opportunities to improve health outcomes. Lack of public trust in the recommendations or perception of undue influence as

[4]Standards of Ethical Conduct for Employees of the Executive Branch, 5 C.F.R. § 2635 (August 7, 1992).

BOX 4-1
Conflict of Interest and Associated Outcomes

Although the published literature focused on clinical practice guidelines, similarities between purpose and desired outcomes allows for broad insight for the DGAC process. Several descriptive reviews have examined conflicts of interest specifically in the context of guideline development, and concluded that conflicts of interest in the development of guidelines may affect outcomes and should be disclosed and managed (Amiri et al., 2014; Choudhry et al., 2002; Cosgrove et al., 2013; IOM, 2009; Mühlhauser and Meyer, 2013). Specific studies of authors' financial relationships with guideline recommendations were found to be limited in the following areas:

- Positive associations between authors' financial conflicts of interest and guideline recommendations. Several studies point toward an association between authors' financial conflicts of interest and recommendations favorable to related drugs or biomedical products (Campsall et al., 2016; George et al., 2014; Norris et al., 2011, 2013).
- Mixed results of author conflicts of interest and voting tendencies. Pham-Kanter (2014) explored author conflicts of interest and voting tendencies in the context of the U.S. Food and Drug Administration (FDA) advisory committees, finding mixed results. Notably, authors with financial ties to a single sponsor, or serving on an advisory board for a single sponsor, were more likely to vote in favor of that sponsor, while authors with financial ties to multiple sponsors were no more likely to vote in favor of those sponsors.
- Mixed impact of industry sponsorship of research. Some reviews have documented industry sponsorship in biomedical and nutrition research being associated with favorable outcomes for the sponsor (Lesser et al., 2007; Ridker and Torres, 2006). However, a systematic review and meta-analysis conducted by Chartres et al. (2016) found that industry-sponsored nutrition studies were more likely to publish outcomes favorable to the sponsor than those not sponsored by industry, but the difference was not significant.

a result of conflicts of interest is another negative outcome. Despite a lack of a formal body of evidence, Box 4-1 highlights some observed associations and the importance of disclosing and managing conflicts of interest.

Although no systematic reviews were identified regarding management strategies on conflict of interest and their associated outcomes, several descriptive studies outlining existing conflict-of-interest policies and proposing best practices were identified (Boyd and Bero, 2006; Boyd et al., 2004, 2012; Mendelson et al., 2011). A thorough examination of conflict-of-interest policies from six organizations,[5] as well as relevant empirical data, found that significant variation existed on how a conflict of interest was defined, how and when it was disclosed, the minimum funding amount requiring report, the time period over which to report, how the disclosure was reviewed, and finally, how the conflict was managed. Still, several improvements for disclosure and management may be possible, as identified in the literature. The review found that all relevant individuals should disclose any potential conflicts of interest. If no conflicts exist, individuals should serve on the committee as planned, and should disclose anything that arises during their course of service that could be a potential conflict (Graham et al., 2015). If a conflict exists, depending on the type (financial or nonfinancial) and severity, these three management strategies may be employed:

1. The individual should not serve on the committee (Rowe et al., 2013).
2. The individual should serve on the committee in a limited capacity, but not participate in decision making or voting regarding the recommendation for which they have a conflict (Guyatt et al., 2010; Neumann et al., 2013).
3. The individual should serve on the committee as long as a counterviewpoint is represented for balance (Viswanathan et al., 2014).

This National Academies committee concludes conflicts of interest—whether actual or perceived cannot always be able to be eliminated entirely on a balanced panel of experts, as conflicts of interest are interpreted to include industrial, professional, political, and cultural influences. Although significant conflicts need to be avoided, some situations may exist where the requisite expertise cannot be found in individuals without conflicts of interest. In these instances, it is necessary to identify, disclose, and manage the influences in question. This National Academies committee concludes USDA and HHS need to develop an explicit policy to address biases and conflicts of interest to be shared with the public. This policy would apply to provisional members being considered for appointment. As discussed previously, individuals who provide input to the advisory committee as consultants or members of a subcommittee would also be assessed for their biases and conflicts of interest.

[5]American College of Chest Physicians, American College of Physicians, American Medical Association, International Committee of Biomedical Journal Editors, Society for Critical Care Medicine, World Health Organization.

Identification

As discussed in Chapter 2, as a federal advisory committee, the current DGAC selection process uses the U.S. Office of Government Ethics' (OGE's) confidential financial disclosure process, including the OGE Form 450 described in Chapter 3. Conflicts of interest for the candidate are taken into consideration, as well as those of the candidate's spouse, minor child, general partner, outside employer, and persons or organizations with whom the candidate is negotiating or has an arrangement for employment. This National Academies committee believes the OGE Form 450 adequately covers financial conflicts of interest, but it did not find any explicit, formal steps for DGAC candidates to disclose nonfinancial conflicts or biases. To enhance transparency, a form should be developed and used for the disclosure of nonfinancial conflicts of interest and biases. Since the OGE only addresses financial conflicts of interest, a form would have to be developed and approved by that office, such as the EPA Form 3110-48 discussed in Chapter 3. A nonfinancial conflict of interest and bias declaration form ought to be designed to capture appropriate professional experiences and relationships relevant to the task for which the individual is being considered. Examples include publications, speeches, testimony, or advisory roles where the individual discussed topics related to the task (see Box 3-3). Additionally, such a form could help identify affiliations or relationships with organizations that could benefit nonfinancially from the outcomes of the task. Once a bias or conflict has been judged to be present, ethics officers ought to try to determine the potential effect of the conflict.

This National Academies committee believes potential biases and conflicts of interest ought to be disclosed to three audiences: the appropriate ethics officers, other members of the specific activity, and to the public. Full disclosure of potential biases and conflicts should be shared with ethics officers via the above-described forms. In addition, disclosure should be made revealing potential sources of conflicts to others serving on the same activity. In the case of the DGAC, provisional members should share their biases and potential sources of conflicts—both financial and nonfinancial—with each other, preferably in a nonpublic administrative meeting. This would allow members to better understand the basis for each other's positions during the advisory committee's work. Finally, this National Academies committee proposes an abstraction of financial conflicts of interest deemed by ethics officials to be significant be shared with the public, including sources of funding, consultancies, and other relationships as appropriate. While it is unclear whether an exemption to the Privacy Act could be made to allow USDA and HHS to require provisional members to share the sources of potential conflicts with the public, this National Academies committee believes that in the spirit of transparency, general information about individual financial conflicts ought to be shared with the public. Provisional DGAC members ought to be willing to share this information publicly at a meeting or through their own means.

This National Academies committee suggests those who have had relationships with industry or advocates in the past 3 years can participate fairly on a panel if the nature of the relationship is incidental to the work of the panel, as it would allow for people with a greater diversity of expertise to potentially serve on the DGAC. Examples of lookback periods ranged from 6 months to 5 years. However, the committee could not identify literature that conclusively supported a specific length of time to consider. Without conclusive evidence about the effect of the length of a lookback period, the committee considered the process to update the *DGA*. Three years equals the amount of time from release of the last edition of the *DGA* to the formation of the next advisory committee. This National Academies committee weighed the potential risks and benefits of various lookback periods and used its collective judgment to agree on 3 years as a reasonable period. Appointment of a diverse DGAC would most clearly be tested if the proposed changes regarding bias and conflict of interest policies are made, and the DGAC composition does not change accordingly.

A detailed description of how biases and conflicts of interest will be identified and judged should be made publicly available as part of a policy on biases and conflicts of interest and ought to be monitored independently by someone not involved in managing the development of the *DGA*. As discussed in Chapter 3, organizations use a variety of structures to assess biases and conflicts of interest. For example, in some instances a steering committee is employed to evaluate and judge the effects of potential conflicts. The executive branch of the federal government relies on its ethics officers and the OGE to make determinations about potential financial conflicts. However, assessment of biases and nonfinancial conflicts are more difficult to make.

Management

Many tools exist to manage conflicts of interest. This National Academies committee recommends that a policy be shared with the public describing (1) a general plan for identifying and resolving biases and conflicts on the whole panel, and (2) plans for managing individuals' specific conflicts, as needed.

Specific to conflicts of interest, exemptions could be applied in instances where the potential conflict is deemed too remote or inconsequential to significantly influence an individual's judgment. Another tool to manage conflicts of interest is the granting of waivers that would allow for varying ranges of participation in the given task depending on the significance and nature of the conflict. Individuals could also choose to sell stock or otherwise divest property deemed a conflict before participation. They could also choose to resign from a potentially disqualifying activity. These and other approaches are often used to mitigate the effect of activities deemed to be actual or perceived conflicts. Changes to the advisory committee's structure could also be adopted to minimize the effect of any undue influence during its work. For example, members with potential conflicts could be excluded from the discussions or recommendations from specific subcommittees or writing groups. Other methods, such as limiting the number of individuals with waivers on the overall advisory committee or on subcommittees, could also be employed.

During the course of an advisory committee's service, other tools can be used to manage both biases and conflicts. A review highlighting any new biases or potential conflicts of interest could be discussed at the beginning of every meeting. When a potential bias is disclosed in relation to an item on the meeting agenda, individuals could be recused from discussions and voting that could be perceived as unduly influencing the work. Specific management plans could be tailored to an individual's personal circumstances. These individualized management plans would explain what specifically was done to try to minimize the effect of any biases or conflicts. These plans ought to remain confidential, and would be reviewed annually by an ethics officer.

Consideration of the benefits and harms related to the management of conflicts of interest is important. Not all conflicts of interest unduly influence a person's actions or decisions while serving on a committee. Although it is important to avoid the perception of conflicts of interest, there are also risks of being too stringent on conflict-of-interest disclosures, such as candidates not wanting to join as a result of an overly burdensome process. Recognizing these risks, how biases and conflicts of interest are managed is critical, and rigorous policies ought to be followed.

Transparent Process for Assessing Bias and Conflict of Interest

The current selection process for the DGAC requires members be screened for financial conflicts of interest and attend ethics training. However, the steps taken during this process are not necessarily clearly delineated or shared with the public. To enhance the process for assessing bias and conflicts of interest, this National Academies committee recommends that the secretaries of USDA and HHS certify that an independent review and assessment of biases and conflicts of interest was conducted. This certification would also include description of any management plans put in place prior to the commencement of the advisory committee's work.

The committee suggests independent reviews be conducted by a federal ethics officer.

Certification provides a level of transparency to the public that biases and conflicts of interest were reviewed prior to the advisory committee's work. A statement should also be made at the conclusion of the work to describe how biases and conflicts of interest were managed at a high level. Such a statement would give the public assurance that the biases and conflicts of interest were appropriately managed throughout the entire course of the advisory committee's work, and that the advisory committee's discussions were not unduly influenced.

Recommendation 3. The secretaries of USDA and HHS should disclose how provisional nominees' biases and conflicts of interest are identified and managed by

a. Creating and publicly posting a policy and form to explicitly disclose financial and nonfinancial biases and conflicts;
b. Developing a management plan for addressing biases and conflicts for the panel as a whole and individuals, as needed;
c. Certifying that a federal ethics officer independently reviewed and judged the advisory committee's biases and conflicts of interest;
d. Documenting how conflicts of interest were managed in the Dietary Guidelines Advisory Committee report.

CONCLUSION

The current selection process for the DGAC can be improved. To that end, this National Academies committee has provided recommendations and suggestions for the secretaries of USDA and HHS to consider to improve transparency and reduce bias. These are generally not radically new ideas, but they could all be implemented to help enhance the integrity of the current process by increasing transparency, identifying the potential for conflict of interest, and appropriately managing these conflicts to minimize bias. As part of an overall, comprehensive review of the process to update the *DGA*, additional findings and recommendations about the selection process may be made as part of this committee's second report.

REFERENCES

Amiri, A. R., K. Kanesalingam, S. Cro, and A. T. Casey. 2014. Does source of funding and conflict of interest influence the outcome and quality of spinal research? *Spine Journal* 14(2):308-314.

Barrow, C. S., and J. W. Conrad. 2006. Assessing the reliability and credibility of industry science and scientists. *Environmental Health Perspectives* 114(2):153-155.

Bindslev, J. B., J. Schroll, P. C. Gotzsche, and A. Lundh. 2013. Underreporting of conflicts of interest in clinical practice guidelines: Cross sectional study. *BMC Medical Ethics* 14:19.

Boyd, E. A., and L. A. Bero. 2006. Improving the use of research evidence in guideline development: 4. Managing conflicts of interests. *Health Research Policy and Systems* 4.

Boyd, E. A., S. Lipton, and L. A. Bero. 2004. Implementation of financial disclosure policies to manage conflicts of interest. *Health Affairs (Millwood)* 23(2):206-214.

Boyd, E. A., E. A. Akl, M. Baumann, J. R. Curtis, M. J. Field, R. Jaeschke, M. Osborne, and H. J. Schunemann. 2012. Guideline funding and conflicts of interest: Article 4 in integrating and coordinating efforts in COPD guideline development. An official ATS/ERS workshop report. *Proceedings of the American Thoracic Society* 9(5):234-242.

Campsall, P., K. Colizza, S. Straus, and H. T. Stelfox. 2016. Financial relationships between organizations that produce clinical practice Guidelines and the biomedical industry: A cross-sectional study. *PLoS Medicine* 13(5):e1002029.

Chartres, N., A. Fabbri, and L. A. Bero. 2016. Association of industry sponsorship with outcomes of nutrition studies: A systematic review and meta-analysis. *JAMA Internal Medicine* 176(12):1769-1777.

Choudhry, N. K., H. T. Stelfox, and A. S. Detsky. 2002. Relationships between authors of clinical practice guidelines and the pharmaceutical industry. *Journal of the American Medical Association* 287(5):612-617.

Cosgrove, L., H. J. Bursztajn, D. R. Erlich, E. E. Wheeler, and A. F. Shaughnessy. 2013. Conflicts of interest and the quality of recommendations in clinical guidelines. *Journal of Evaluation in Clinical Practice* 19(4):674-681.

DOL (U.S. Department of Labor). 2015. Advisory Board on Toxic Substances and Worker Health notice of comment period. *Federal Register* 80(199):62111-62113.

EPA (U.S. Environmental Protection Agency). 2014. *Invitation for public comment on the list of candidates for the EPA science advisory board chemical assessment advisory committee augmented for benzo[a]pyrene review* https://yosemite.epa.gov/sab/sabproduct.nsf/0/4DCFD0E5F45A8CAD85257B65005B17C8/$File/List%20of%20candidates%20with%20Biosketch%209-18-2014.pdf (accessed October 5, 2017).

GAO (U.S. Government Accountability Office). 2016. *Health care advisory committees.* http://www.gao.gov/about/hcac/index.html (accessed October 5, 2017).

George, J. N., S. K. Vesely, and S. H. Woolf. 2014. Conflicts of interest and clinical recommendations: Comparison of two concurrent clinical practice guidelines for primary immune thrombocytopenia developed by different methods. *American Journal of Medical Quality* 29(1):53-60.

Gessner, B. D., P. Duclos, D. DeRoeck, and E. A. S. Nelson. 2010. Informing decision makers: Experience and process of 15 national immunization technical advisory groups. *Vaccine* 28(Suppl 1):A1-A5.

Graham, T., P. Alderson, and T. Stokes. 2015. Managing conflicts of interest in the UK National Institute for Health and Care Excellence (NICE) clinical guidelines programme: Qualitative study. *PLoS ONE* 10(3):e0122313.

Gummalla, S. 2016 (unpublished). *Comments presented at USDA* Dietary Guidelines for Americans *listening sessions: American Frozen Food Institute.* Washington, DC, February 19, 2016.

Guyatt, G., E. A. Akl, J. Hirsh, C. Kearon, M. Crowther, D. Gutterman, S. Z. Lewis, I. Nathanson, R. Jaeschke, and H. Schünemann. 2010. The vexing problem of guidelines and conflict of interest: A potential solution. *Annals of Internal Medicine* 152(11):738-741.

HHS (U.S. Department of Health and Human Services). 2015. *National Vaccine Advisory Committee charter.* https://www.hhs.gov/nvpo/nvac/charter/index.html (accessed October 5, 2017).

HHS. 2016. *Physician-Focused Payment Model Technical Advisory Committee charter.* https://aspe.hhs.gov/charter-physician-focused-payment-model-technical-advisory-committee (accessed October 5, 2017).

IOM (Institute of Medicine). 2009. *Conflict of interest in medical research, education, and practice.* Washington, DC: The National Academies Press.

IOM. 2011. *Clinical practice guidelines we can trust.* Washington, DC: The National Academies Press.

Khalil, B., K. Aung, and I. A. Mansi. 2012. Reporting potential conflicts of interest among authors of professional medical societies' guidelines. *Southern Medical Journal* 105(8):411-415.

Lesser, L. I., C. B. Ebbeling, M. Goozner, D. Wypij, and D. S. Ludwig. 2007. Relationship between funding source and conclusion among nutrition-related scientific articles. *PLoS Medicine* 4(1):e5.

Maitin-Shepard, M. 2016 (unpublished). *Comments presented at USDA* Dietary Guidelines for Americans *listening sessions: American Cancer Society/American Cancer Society Cancer Action Network.* Washington, DC, February 19, 2016.

Mendelson, T. B., M. Meltzer, E. G. Campbell, A. L. Caplan, and J. N. Kirkpatrick. 2011. Conflicts of interest in cardiovascular clinical practice guidelines. *Archives of Internal Medicine* 171(6):577-584.

Mozaffarian, D. 2016 (unpublished). *Comments presented at USDA* Dietary Guidelines for Americans *listening sessions.* Washington, DC, February 19, 2016.

Mühlhauser, I., and G. Meyer. 2013. Evidence base in guideline generation in diabetes. *Diabetologia* 56(6):1201-1209.

Neumann, I., R. Karl, A. Rajpal, E. A. Akl, and G. H. Guyatt. 2013. Experiences with a novel policy for managing conflicts of interest of guideline developers: A descriptive qualitative study. *Chest* 144(2):398-404.

NIH (National Institutes of Health). 2016. *Biosketch format pages, instructions and samples.* http://grants.nih.gov/grants/forms/biosketch-instructions-Forms-D.docx (accessed October 5, 2017).

Norris, S. L., H. K. Holmer, L. A. Ogden, and B. U. Burda. 2011. Conflict of interest in clinical practice guideline development: A systematic review. *PLoS ONE* 6(10):e25153.

Norris, S. L., H. K. Holmer, L. A. Ogden, B. U. Burda, and R. Fu. 2013. Conflicts of interest among authors of clinical practice guidelines for glycemic control in type 2 diabetes mellitus. *PLoS ONE* 8(10):e75284.

Pham-Kanter, G. 2014. Revisiting financial conflicts of interest in FDA advisory committees. *The Milbank Quarterly* 92(3):446-470.

Ridker, P., and J. Torres. 2006. Reported outcomes in major cardiovascular clinical trials funded by for-profit and not-for-profit organizations: 2000-2005. *Journal of the American Medical Association* 295(19):2270-2274.

Rowe, S., N. Alexander, F. M. Clydesdale, R. S. Applebaum, S. Atkinson, R. M. Black, J. T. Dwyer, E. Hentges, N. A. Higley, M. Lefevre, J. R. Lupton, S. A. Miller, D. L. Tancredi, C. M. Weaver, C. E. Woteki, and E. Wedral. 2009. Funding food science and nutrition research: Financial conflicts and scientific integrity. *American Journal of Clinical Nutrition* 89(5):1285-1291.

Rowe, S., N. Alexander, C. M. Weaver, J. T. Dwyer, C. Drew, R. S. Applebaum, S. Atkinson, F. M. Clydesdale, E. Hentges, N. A. Higley, and M. E. Westring. 2013. How experts are chosen to inform public policy: Can the process be improved? *Health Policy* 112(3):172-178.

Schünemann, H. J., A. Fretheim, and A. D. Oxman. 2006. Improving the use of research evidence in guideline development: 1. Guidelines for guidelines. *Health Research Policy and Systems* 4(13).

Schünemann, H. J., L. A. Al-Ansary, F. Forland, S. Kersten, J. Komulainen, I. B. Kopp, F. Macbeth, S. M. Phillips, C. Robbins, P. Van der Wees, and A. Qaseem. 2015. Guidelines international network: Principles for disclosure of interests and management of conflicts in Guidelines. *Annals of Internal Medicine* 163(7):548-553.

Tibau, A., P. L. Bedard, A. Srikanthan, J. L. Ethier, F. E. Vera-Badillo, A. J. Templeton, A. Ocana, B. Seruga, A. Barnadas, and E. Amir. 2015. Author financial conflicts of interest, industry funding, and clinical practice guidelines for anticancer drugs. *Journal of Clinical Oncology* 33(1):100-106.

USDA/HHS (U.S. Department of Agriculture/U.S. Department of Health and Human Services). 2016a (unpublished). Dietary Guidelines for Americans: *Process brief, sections 1–3.* Prepared for the Committee to Review the Process to Update the *Dietary Guidelines for Americans.*

USDA/HHS. 2016b (unpublished). *HMD follow-up questions for USDA* Response to Committee to Review the Process to Update the *Dietary Guidelines for Americans.*

Viswanathan, M., T. S. Carey, S. E. Belinson, E. Berliner, S. M. Chang, E. Graham, J.-M. Guise, S. Ip, M. A. Maglione, D. C. McCrory, M. McPheeters, S. J. Newberry, P. Sista, and C. M. White. 2014. A proposed approach may help systematic reviews retain needed expertise while minimizing bias from nonfinancial conflicts of interest. *Journal of Clinical Epidemiology* 67(11):1229-1238.

Willett, W. 2016 (unpublished). *Invited perspectives: What two recommendations would you make to USDA/HHS related to the Dietary Guidelines Advisory Committee selection process.* Presentation to the Committee to Review the Process to Update the *Dietary Guidelines for Americans.*

5

A Continuously Learning Selection Process

The Dietary Guidelines Advisory Committee (DGAC) selection process comprises a set of steps designed to help attain specific goals. When implemented in an environment of high-velocity change, a process may not always continue to yield desired results. It will be important for the U.S. Department of Agriculture (USDA) and the U.S. Department of Health and Human Services (HHS) to dynamically improve the DGAC selection process to achieve desired results over time.

A VISION FOR CONTINUOUS QUALITY IMPROVEMENT

Sustained, optimal performance is the product of systematic quality improvement activities. These activities address outcomes such as cycle time, efficiency, defects, duplication, and waste (Deming, 1982; Sehwail and DeYong, 2003; Womack et al., 1990). While these methods and tools were created in manufacturing environments, their use in services and policy are now well established in many sectors, including health care (Berwick et al., 2008; Taner et al., 2007). Quality improvement is indispensable to continuously learning systems. It helps an organization drive toward positive change, and it also contributes to enhanced adoption, use, and trust from a variety of stakeholders. High-performing processes also help to deeply embed quality improvement in an organization's management systems and cultures.

The field of quality improvement has undergone a transformation in response to changes needing to be made in shorter, faster time intervals.

The focus has shifted from identifying, fixing, and improving processes in an ad hoc manner, to dynamically learning and adapting. One well-recognized and extensively used approach of quality improvement in the private and public sectors is the Plan-Do-Study-Act cycle. It employs iterative cycles of design, execution, measurement, and evaluation. The first step of the cycle is planning. This involves key stakeholder engagement to help design a clear statement of objectives and develop a detailed implementation plan. Actively seeking input from stakeholders is critical to developing a product relevant to the end users. Also important to the planning phase is development of actionable metrics to evaluate performance and achievement of objectives. The second step of the cycle—"do"—implements the intervention and activates the data collection process, including notation of problems and observations. The context surrounding each change is also documented in this phase. "Study" is the third step of the cycle and involves the timely analysis of data collected to quantify performance against objectives. The final step of the cycle is to "act" on the data-driven insights by identifying the next opportunities for improvement and repeating the cycle.

Ideally, the *Dietary Guidelines for Americans* (*DGA*) would engage in a continuous process improvement system, beginning with the DGAC selection process. The DGAC selection process has been modified over time but not as a consequence of a proactive, disciplined quality improvement process. As a result, little data currently exist to evaluate the effectiveness of the DGAC selection process. There are many opportunities to make the DGAC selection process more evidence based. This National Academies of Sciences, Engineering, and Medicine (the National Academies) committee believes the aforementioned attributes of quality improvement are critical to improving the DGAC selection process. A system for continuous quality improvement can have significant benefits, but takes time and commitment to develop.

Recommendation 4. The secretaries of USDA and HHS should adopt a system for continuous process improvement to enhance outcomes and performance of the Dietary Guidelines Advisory Committee selection process.

APPLICATION TO THE DGAC SELECTION PROCESS

This National Academies committee sought to base its recommendations on objective science, but found little evidence to objectively assess the DGAC selection process. To measure how effective or trustworthy the selection process is, and where opportunities exist to improve, a concerted effort needs to be made. Actionable measures to evaluate the DGAC selection process need to be created. Data have to be identified and baseline measurements taken. Plans for implementation and evaluation have to be made. A commitment to a culture of change is needed to continuously learn, respond, and adapt.

Of critical importance to adopting a continuous quality improvement system is stakeholder engagement. Stakeholders of the *DGA* include the general public, the government, industry, and issue-specific advocates. Specific to the DGAC selection process, as discussed in Chapter 4, it will be important to offer interested parties as many opportunities as practicable to provide input. Active stakeholder engagement can help engender trust in a balanced and effective DGAC.

Recognizing that changes to the DGAC selection process will not be immediate, this National Academies committee suggests actions to be taken in the short term, focused at three levels: the overall selection process, the advisory committee's structure, and the advisory committee itself.

Overall Selection Process

The overall selection process ought to be decomposed and each element be evaluated for its current effect on stakeholder trust and perceptions of integrity. A key hypothesis to be tested is that changes made to enhance transparency of the selection process actually result in greater public trust and insight as to how nominees are considered for appointment to the DGAC. The recommendations in Chapter 4, such as the use of a third party to narrow the pool of candidates, addition of public comment periods, and development of strategies to identify and manage biases and conflicts of interest, all ought to be studied for their ability to add value. The criteria for selection also ought to be evaluated and tailored as needed. It will be important to capture both favorable and adverse unintended consequences of such changes and for the process to react accordingly.

The effects of detailed decisions made while designing the selection process also need to be reviewed. For example, what are the most relevant materials to collect during the nominations process? What oversight processes are in place for ensuring implementation of the process is fair and just? Is there a marked advantage to collecting full bias and conflict-of-interest information from all candidates before a slate of members is proposed? These questions and others ought to be prioritized and considered over time.

To test hypotheses, interventions and outcomes first need to be measured and baseline data have to be collected, but trust is a difficult outcome to measure. Success of the *DGA* relies on the programs and health professionals (e.g., individual dieticians, physicians) responsible for disseminating the guidelines. The definitive measures of trust in the *DGA* therefore are (1) the percent of these programs' and health professionals' familiarity and buy-in, and ultimately (2) the percent of the public adhering to the advice. Although these would be complex to measure, they could be longer-term measures to assess based on initial measurements by academic centers and others.

Additionally, this National Academies committee could not develop a litmus test to gauge outcomes midcourse. A number of intermediate outcomes could be developed. For example, data could be collected through surveys and focus groups using carefully crafted questionnaires asking members of the public if they believe the process is fair and if they are confident in the implementation and results. While other less descriptive assessments could be made, they are also important to capture, such as the numbers and types of public comments received. Simulation models could also be built to gauge the potential effect of specific interventions on the efficiency and effectiveness of the process.

Advisory Committee Structure

A second level of evaluation to consider is the advisory committee's structure. The structure includes the advisory committee's operating procedures and the roles of members, as well as the effect of biases and conflicts of interest. These factors can all influence whether a wide range of viewpoints and expertise are considered during deliberations.

An assessment of the DGAC's operating procedures could be warranted. By tradition, the DGAC scientific report has been a consensus document. However, future DGACs may want to discuss the value in allowing members to post an explanation of why they do not agree with a particular conclusion. This could be done in a number of ways, such as issuing minority opinions and publishing unresolved questions with conflicting data as needed. Alternatively, assessments could be warranted to identify whether voting is an effective way of letting the public know what conclusions are made and by what margins.

Examples and evidence are also needed to identify the effect of different advisory committee structures. Whether having the advisory committee comprise members of voting and nonvoting status leads to inclusion of a broader range of viewpoints and expertise ought to be studied. As discussed in Chapter 4, the effects of various external inputs to the advisory committee, such as consultants, non-DGAC members on subcommittees, and invited expert speakers, would also be important to review. Future DGACs ought to reflect on the learnings from assessments of varying committee compositions.

An evaluation of the potential effect of the DGAC's composition and structure could verify that the process does engender the fair sharing of opinions. To measure the extent to which diverse opinions are considered, it would be beneficial to hear from the members themselves, potentially through interviews or surveys.

The effects of various tools to manage biases and conflicts of interest are also critical and need to be evaluated. Because of the complexity inherent in characterizing and managing conflicts of interest, and the current variation in policies, it is not surprising that comprehensive intervention studies are not available. However, strengthening the evidence base is critical to further understanding of how conflict-of-interest policies affect the development of advisory committees and their subsequent recommendations. A number of areas have been identified where additional research could strengthen and improve management of conflict of interest, including

- identifying relationships and their associated level of risk of conflicts of interest arising,
- characterizing policies that achieve the desired outcome of reducing the risk of bias and reducing the appearance of bias, and
- monitoring any unintended negative consequences of policy implementation in order to continue to allow organizations to manage conflicts in the most effective way possible (IOM, 2009).

This National Academies committee identified several key components of a comprehensive study on conflict of interest when considering additional research to better inform selection processes:

- Clearly define conflicts of interest and the potential types and strata of disqualifying activities.
- Identify the effects of a procedural intervention or strategy to manage biases and conflicts of interest (e.g., the removal of individuals from voting on issues where there may be a conflict of interest).
- Discuss any unique considerations for the specific population or type of guidelines in consideration (e.g., the relative availability of nonconflicted subject-matter experts).
- Describe the specific effect of bias and conflict of interest depending on what is being considered (e.g., a person whose research strongly favors a certain point of view would have more relevant biases when considering an alternative point of view).
- Evaluate findings tied to outcomes of interest, including any reduction in the number of recommendations possibly influenced

by advisory committee members' conflicts of interest or number of perceived conflicts. A correlated outcome of interest would be an increase in public trust; however, it is important to recognize that trustworthiness is multifactorial and is more than an assessment of real or perceived conflicts of interest.

Advisory Committee Functions

Specific to the DGAC selection process, evaluations related to how the advisory committee functions also ought to be conducted, such as examining the effectiveness of the leadership team and, as applicable, the roles of a chair and vice chair. Potential benefits of facilitators and other outside collaborators could also be reviewed as additional support in balancing perspectives and potential biases throughout advisory committee deliberations. Consultants could bring techniques, methods, and technologies that can help identify biases and mitigate them. More research is also needed on the effect of different potential biases on various recommendations. For example, are there particular types of recommendations that would be more or less susceptible to bias? Different methods to mitigate such biases are needed to assess how best to drive improvements at the level of the advisory committee.

CONCLUSION

The DGAC selection process needs to dynamically evolve and improve. A system needs to be developed so improvements are grounded in evidence. Lessons should be learned from each cycle and integrated into future selection processes. Best practices from other advisory committees and bodies of literature should also be incorporated. However, a continuous process improvement system requires a long-term commitment and resources to appropriately collect data and measure change. It will be important to measure not only improvements in the selection process, but also any unintended adverse consequences. Proven continuous process improvements can help improve the integrity of the DGAC selection process and merit the public's trust.

REFERENCES

Berwick, D. M., T. W. Nolan, and J. Whittington. 2008. The triple aim: Care, health, and cost. *Health Affairs* 27(3):759-769.

Deming, W. E. 1982. *Quality, productivity, and competitive position*. Cambridge, MA: Massachussets Institute of Technology.

IOM (Institute of Medicine). 2009. *Conflict of interest in medical research, education, and practice*. Washington, DC: The National Academies Press.

Sehwail, L., and C. DeYong. 2003. Six sigma in health care. *Leadership in Health Services* 16(4):1-5.

Taner, M. T., B. Sezen, and J. Antony. 2007. An overview of six sigma applications in healthcare industry. *International Journal of Health Care Quality Assurance* 20(4):329-340.

Womack, J. P., D. T. Jones, and D. Roos. 1990. *The machine that changed the world*. New York: Free Press.

Appendix A

Literature Search Strategy for "Conflict of Interest"

This National Academies of Sciences, Engineering, and Medicine (the National Academies) committee recognizes the importance of considering conflicts of interest in contributing to and detracting from the public's trust in the development of guidelines. To supplement previous evidence reviews and to identify additional resources for consideration, the committee conducted a focused literature review guided by the following preliminary questions:

1. How are conflicts of interest managed in guideline development and/or in advisory committees? This may include but is not limited to the following:
    a. Evidence review
    b. Expert group or advisory committee formation
    c. Translation to recommendations or practice
    d. Project funding
2. Are there any conflict-of-interest practices specific to nutrition or diet research and guidelines?

The main finding was significant variation of conflict-of-interest policies and practices across organizations and within guideline development processes, and limited empirical evidence linking these policies and practices to desired outcomes. This search was not intended to be a comprehensive review, but rather to identify relevant and recent publications for consideration.

SEARCH TERMS

A keyword search was run through Web of Science, PubMed, and Scopus. Keywords included *conflict of interest, conflicts of interest, conflicting interest, competing interest, financial conflicts, commercial conflicts, funding, disclosure, guideline, guidelines, guidelines as topic, practice guidelines, committee, committees, advisory committee, committee membership, review literature, organizational policy, policy, policies, nutritional policy,* and *industry*. The search was restricted to English language.

SCREENING

More than 800 unique articles were found, 62 of which met inclusion criteria of describing or managing conflicts of interest in the development of guidelines and advisory committees. The narrow focus of the search excluded conflicts of interest in areas not directly applicable (e.g., conflicts of interest in human subject research), while noting that many articles would be relevant to this National Academies committee's second report. Two reviewers independently screened selected titles and abstracts for inclusion in the full-text review. An additional scan of the reference lists of relevant publications and previous Institute of Medicine publications (IOM, 2009, 2011) led to the identification and ad-hoc inclusion of additional articles. Some articles were determined not to be relevant and were excluded based on the full-text review. In total, 62 references were included and are listed below.

REFERENCES

Akl, E. A., P. El-Hachem, H. Abou-Haidar, I. Neumann, H. J. Schunemann, and G. H. Guyatt. 2014. Considering intellectual, in addition to financial, conflicts of interest proved important in a clinical practice guideline: A descriptive study. *Journal of Clinical Epidemiology* 67(11):1222-1228.

Amiri, A. R., K. Kanesalingam, S. Cro, and A. T. Casey. 2014. Does source of funding and conflict of interest influence the outcome and quality of spinal research? *Spine Journal* 14(2):308-314.

Barrow, C. S., and J. W. Conrad. 2006. Assessing the reliability and credibility of industry science and scientists. *Environmental Health Perspectives* 114(2):153-155.

Bero, L. 2014. What is in a name? Nonfinancial influences on the outcomes of systematic reviews and guidelines. *Journal of Clinical Epidemiology* 67(11):1239-1241.

Billi, J. E., B. Eigel, W. H. Montgomery, V. M. Nadkarni, and M. F. Hazinski. 2005. Management of conflict of interest issues in the activities of the American Heart Association Emergency Cardiovascular Care Committee, 2000-2005. *Circulation* 112(24 Suppl.):IV204-IV205.

Bindslev, J. B., J. Schroll, P. C. Gotzsche, and A. Lundh. 2013. Underreporting of conflicts of interest in clinical practice guidelines: Cross sectional study. *BMC Medical Ethics* 14:19.

Boyd, E. A., and L. A. Bero. 2006. Improving the use of research evidence in guideline development: 4. Managing conflicts of interests. *Health Research Policy and Systems* 4.

Boyd, E. A., S. Lipton, and L. A. Bero. 2004. Implementation of financial disclosure policies to manage conflicts of interest. *Health Affairs (Millwood)* 23(2):206-214.

Boyd, E. A., E. A. Akl, M. Baumann, J. R. Curtis, M. J. Field, R. Jaeschke, M. Osborne, and H. J. Schunemann. 2012. Guideline funding and conflicts of interest: Article 4 in integrating and coordinating efforts in COPD guideline development. An official ATS/ERS workshop report. *Proceedings of the American Thoracic Society* 9(5):234-242.

Campsall, P., K. Colizza, S. Straus, and H. T. Stelfox. 2016. Financial relationships between organizations that produce clinical practice guidelines and the biomedical industry: A cross-sectional study. *PLoS Medicine* 13(5):e1002029.

Chartres, N., A. Fabbri, and L. A. Bero. 2016. Association of industry sponsorship with outcomes of nutrition studies: A systematic review and meta-analysis. *JAMA Internal Medicine* 176(12):1769-1777.

Choudhry, N. K., H. T. Stelfox, and A. S. Detsky. 2002. Relationships between authors of clinical practice guidelines and the pharmaceutical industry. *Journal of the American Medical Association* 287(5):612-617.

Cosgrove, L., H. J. Bursztajn, D. R. Erlich, E. E. Wheeler, and A. F. Shaughnessy. 2013. Conflicts of interest and the quality of recommendations in clinical guidelines. *Journal of Evaluation in Clinical Practice* 19(4):674-681.

Eccles, M. P., J. M. Grimshaw, P. Shekelle, H. J. Schunemann, and S. Woolf. 2012. Developing clinical practice guidelines: Target audiences, identifying topics for guidelines, guideline group composition and functioning and conflicts of interest. *Implementation Science* 7:60.

Esposito, K., A. Ceriello, S. Genovese, and D. Giugliano. 2014. Cardiovascular guidelines: Separate career may help attenuate controversy. *Cardiovascular Diabetology* 13(1):66.

Evans, I. 2002. Conflict of interest: The importance of potential. *Science and Engineering Ethics* 8(3):393-396.

FDA (U.S. Food and Drug Administration). 2014. *Guidance for the public, FDA advisory committee members, and FDA staff: Public availability of advisory committee members' financial interest information and waivers.* Silver Spring, MD: U.S. Food and Drug Administration. http://www.fda.gov/RegulatoryInformation/Guidances/ucm122045.htm (accessed October 5, 2017).

George, J. N., S. K. Vesely, and S. H. Woolf. 2014. Conflicts of interest and clinical recommendations: Comparison of two concurrent clinical practice guidelines for primary immune thrombocytopenia developed by different methods. *American Journal of Medical Quality* 29(1):53-60.

Gessner, B. D., P. Duclos, D. DeRoeck, and E. A. S. Nelson. 2010. Informing decision makers: Experience and process of 15 national immunization technical advisory groups. *Vaccine* 28(Suppl 1):A1-A5.

Gibbons, R. J., S. Smith, and E. Antman. 2003. American College of Cardiology/American Heart Association clinical practice guidelines: Part I. Where do they come from? *Circulation* 107(23):2979-2986.

Glodé, E. R. 2002. Advising under the influence?: Conflicts of interest among FDA advisory committee members. *Food and Drug Law Journal* 57(2):293-322.

Graham, T., P. Alderson, and T. Stokes. 2015. Managing conflicts of interest in the UK National Institute for Health and Care Excellence (NICE) clinical guidelines programme: Qualitative study. *PLoS ONE* 10(3):e0122313.

Grisso, T., E. Baldwin, P. D. Blanck, M. J. Rotheram-Borus, N. R. Schooler, and T. Thompson. 1991. Standards in research: APA's mechanism for monitoring the challenges. *American Psychologist* 46(7):758-766.

Guyatt, G., E. A. Akl, J. Hirsh, C. Kearon, M. Crowther, D. Gutterman, S. Z. Lewis, I. Nathanson, R. Jaeschke, and H. Schünemann. 2010. The vexing problem of guidelines and conflict of interest: A potential solution. *Annals of Internal Medicine* 152(11):738-741.

Haines, I. E., and I. N. Olver. 2008. Are self-regulation and declaration of conflict of interest still the benchmark for relationships between physicians and industry? *Medical Journal of Australia* 189(5):263-266.

Holloway, R. G., C. J. Mooney, T. S. D. Getchius, W. S. Edlund, and J. O. Miyasaki. 2008. Invited article: Conflicts of interest for authors of American Academy of Neurology clinical practice guidelines. *Neurology* 71(1):57-63.

IOM (Institute of Medicine). 2009. *Conflict of interest in medical research, education, and practice.* Washington, DC: The National Academies Press.

IOM. 2011. *Clinical practice guidelines we can trust*. Washington, DC: The National Academies Press.

Jones, D. J., A. N. Barkun, Y. Lu, R. Enns, P. Sinclair, M. Martel, I. Gralnek, M. Bardou, E. J. Kuipers, and J. Sung. 2012. Conflicts of interest ethics: Silencing expertise in the development of international clinical practice guidelines. *Annals of Internal Medicine* 156(11):809-816.

Kassirer, J. P. 2009. Commentary: Disclosure's failings: What is the alternative? *Academic Medicine* 84(9):1180-1181.

Khalil, B., K. Aung, and I. A. Mansi. 2012. Reporting potential conflicts of interest among authors of professional medical societies' guidelines. *Southern Medical Journal* 105(8):411-415.

Lesser, L. I., C. B. Ebbeling, M. Goozner, D. Wypij, and D. S. Ludwig. 2007. Relationship between funding source and conclusion among nutrition-related scientific articles. *PLoS Medicine* 4(1):e5.

MacKenzie, R., and W. Rogers. 2015. Potential conflict of interest and bias in the RACGP's smoking cessation guidelines: Are GPs provided with the best advice on smoking cessation for their patients? *Public Health Ethics* 8(3):319-331.

Mendelson, T. B., M. Meltzer, E. G. Campbell, A. L. Caplan, and J. N. Kirkpatrick. 2011. Conflicts of interest in cardiovascular clinical practice guidelines. *Archives of Internal Medicine* 171(6):577-584.

Mühlhauser, I. 2010. From authority recommendations to fact-sheets—A future for guidelines. *Diabetologia* 53(11):2285-2288.

Mühlhauser, I., and G. Meyer. 2013. Evidence base in guideline generation in diabetes. *Diabetologia* 56(6):1201-1209.

Nathanson, I. 2013. Guidelines and conflicts: A new twist. *Chest* 144(4):1087-1089.

Neumann, I., E. A. Akl, M. Valdes, S. Bravo, S. Araos, V. Kairouz, H. Schünemann, and G. H. Guyatt. 2013a. Low anonymous voting compliance with the novel policy for managing conflicts of interest implemented in the 9th version of the American College of Chest Physicians antithrombotic guidelines. *Chest* 144(4):1111-1116.

Neumann, I., R. Karl, A. Rajpal, E. A. Akl, and G. H. Guyatt. 2013b. Experiences with a novel policy for managing conflicts of interest of guideline developers: A descriptive qualitative study. *Chest* 144(2):398-404.

Newton, A., F. Lloyd-Williams, H. Bromley, and S. Capewell. 2016. Food for thought? Potential conflicts of interest in academic experts advising government and charities on dietary policies. *BMC Public Health* 16(1):735.

Norris, S. L., H. K. Holmer, L. A. Ogden, and B. U. Burda. 2011. Conflict of interest in clinical practice guideline development: A systematic review. *PLoS ONE* 6(10):e25153.

Norris, S. L., H. K. Holmer, B. U. Burda, L. A. Ogden, and R. Fu. 2012a. Conflict of interest policies for organizations producing a large number of clinical practice guidelines. *PLoS ONE* 7(5):e37413.

Norris, S. L., H. K. Holmer, L. A. Ogden, S. S. Selph, and R. Fu. 2012b. Conflict of interest disclosures for clinical practice guidelines in the national guideline clearinghouse. *PLoS ONE* 7(11):e47343.

Norris, S. L., H. K. Holmer, L. A. Ogden, B. U. Burda, and R. Fu. 2013. Conflicts of interest among authors of clinical practice guidelines for glycemic control in type 2 diabetes mellitus. *PLoS ONE* 8(10):e75284.

Pham-Kanter, G. 2014. Revisiting financial conflicts of interest in FDA advisory committees. *Milbank Quarterly* 92(3):446-470.

Qaseem, A., F. Forland, F. Macbeth, G. Ollenschlager, S. Phillips, and P. van der Wees. 2012. Guidelines international network: Toward international standards for clinical practice guidelines. *Annals of Internal Medicine* 156(7):525-531.

Reardon, R., and S. Haldeman. 2008. Self-study of values, beliefs, and conflict of interest: The bone and joint decade 2000–2010 task force on neck pain and its associated disorders. *Spine* 33(4 Suppl):S24-S32.

Ridker, P., and J. Torres. 2006. Reported outcomes in major cardiovascular clinical trials funded by for-profit and not-for-profit organizations: 2000–2005. *Journal of the American Medical Association* 295(19):2270-2274.

Riechelmann, R. P., L. Wang, A. O'Carroll, and M. K. Krzyzanowska. 2007. Disclosure of conflicts of interest by authors of clinical trials and editorials in oncology. *Journal of Clinical Oncology* 25(29):4642-4647.

Rosenberg-Yunger, Z. R. S., and A. M. Bayoumi. 2014. Transparency in Canadian public drug advisory committees. *Health Policy* 118(2):255-263.

Rowe, S., N. Alexander, F. M. Clydesdale, R. S. Applebaum, S. Atkinson, R. M. Black, J. T. Dwyer, E. Hentges, N. A. Higley, M. Lefevre, J. R. Lupton, S. A. Miller, D. L. Tancredi, C. M. Weaver, C. E. Woteki, and E. Wedral. 2009. Funding food science and nutrition research: Financial conflicts and scientific integrity. *American Journal of Clinical Nutrition* 89(5):1285-1291.

Rowe, S., N. Alexander, C. M. Weaver, J. T. Dwyer, C. Drew, R. S. Applebaum, S. Atkinson, F. M. Clydesdale, E. Hentges, N. A. Higley, M. E. Westring, and International Life Sciences Institute. 2013. How experts are chosen to inform public policy: Can the process be improved? *Health Policy* 112(3):172-178.

Schroter, S., J. Morris, S. Chaudhry, R. Smith, and H. Barratt. 2004. Does the type of competing interest statement affect readers' perceptions of the credibility of research? Randomised trial. *British Medical Journal* 328(7442):742-743.

Schünemann, H. J., A. Fretheim, and A. D. Oxman. 2006. Improving the use of research evidence in guideline development: 1. Guidelines for guidelines. *Health Research Policy and Systems* 4(13).

Schünemann, H. J., M. Osborne, J. Moss, C. Manthous, G. Wagner, L. Sicilian, J. Ohar, S. McDermott, L. Lucas, and R. Jaeschke. 2009. An official American Thoracic Society policy statement: Managing conflict of interest in professional societies. *American Journal of Respiratory and Critical Care Medicine* 180(6):564-580.

Smith, J. C., D. E. Snider, and L. K. Pickering. 2009. Immunization policy development in the United States: The role of the advisory committee on immunization practices. *Annals of Internal Medicine* 150(1):45-49.

Steinbrook, R. 2007. Guidance for guidelines. *New England Journal of Medicine* 356(4):331-333.

Tattersall, M. H. N., and I. N. Olver. 1999. Conflict of interests and advisory committees. *International Journal of Pharmaceutical Medicine* 13(6):325-328.

Tibau, A., P. L. Bedard, A. Srikanthan, J. L. Ethier, F. E. Vera-Badillo, A. J. Templeton, A. Ocana, B. Seruga, A. Barnadas, and E. Amir. 2015. Author financial conflicts of interest, industry funding, and clinical practice guidelines for anticancer drugs. *Journal of Clinical Oncology* 33(1):100-106.

Viswanathan, M., T. S. Carey, S. E. Belinson, E. Berliner, S. M. Chang, E. Graham, J.-M. Guise, S. Ip, M. A. Maglione, D. C. McCrory, M. McPheeters, S. J. Newberry, P. Sista, and C. M. White. 2014. A proposed approach may help systematic reviews retain needed expertise while minimizing bias from nonfinancial conflicts of interest. *Journal of Clinical Epidemiology* 67(11):1229-1238.

Wood, S. F., and J. K. Mador. 2013. Uncapping conflict of interest? *Science* 340(6137):1172-1173.

Yank, V., D. Rennie, and L. A. Bero. 2007. Financial ties and concordance between results and conclusions in meta-analyses: Retrospective cohort study. *British Medical Journal* 335(7631):1202-1205.

Appendix B

Public Workshop Agendas and Comments

The committee held two open sessions, on September 1, 2016, via WebEx and on October 17, 2016, in Washington, DC. Agendas can be found below.

September 1, 2016
WebEx

10:00–11:00	**Understanding the Committee's Charge: A Discussion with the Sponsor**
	Introductory remarks, Rob Russell, Chair
	Statement from the U.S. Department of Agriculture (USDA) and the U.S. Department of Health and Human Services (HHS)
	    Angie Tagtow and Eve Essery Stoody, USDA
	    Don Wright, HHS
	Discussion and Q&A

October 17, 2016
500 Fifth Street, NW, Room 101
Washington, DC

8:30	**Welcome and Introductory Remarks** Rob Russell, Chair

8:35 **Discussion of Current *Dietary Guidelines for Americans* (*DGA*) and Dietary Guidelines Advisory Committee Processes**

- Opening remarks, Angie Tagtow, USDA
- Advisory committee selection and process, Eve Essery Stoody, USDA
- Nutrition Evidence Library systematic review methodology, Julie Obbagy, USDA
- Updating the *DGA*, Kellie Casavale, HHS

10:00 **Approaches to Biases and Conflicts of Interest**

How would you suggest minimizing conflicts of interest and "eliminating bias" while preserving a wide range of viewpoints?

- Peter Jacobson, University of Michigan
- Sheldon Greenfield, University of California, Irvine
- Quyen Ngo-Metzger, Agency for Healthcare Research and Quality

11:20 **Perspectives**

What two recommendations would you make to USDA/HHS related to the dietary guidelines advisory committee selection process?

- Walter Willett, Harvard University (remote)
- Richard Black, independent consultant (remote)

12:10 **Public Comments**

1:00 **Adjourn**

Public comments were made in person on October 17, 2016, and received online from the following individuals and groups in response to the question "How can the advisory committee selection process be improved to provide more transparency, eliminate bias, and include committee members with a range of viewpoints?":

American Bakers Association
American Cancer Society and American Cancer Society Cancer Action Network
American Frozen Food Institute
Atkins Nutritionals, Inc.
Center for Science in the Public Interest
Grocery Manufacturers of America

Infant Nutrition Council of America
National Milk Producers Federation
North American Meat Institute
Physicians Committee for Responsible Medicine
The Sugar Association
Union of Concerned Scientists

David Allison
Nils Hoernle
Richard Kahn
Lani Kroemer
Lucrecia Rodrigues
John L. Sievenpiper

Appendix C

Committee Member and Staff Biographies

COMMITTEE MEMBERS

Robert M. Russell, M.D. (*Chair*), is professor emeritus of Medicine and Nutrition at Tufts University. Dr. Russell has served on many national and international advisory boards, including the U.S. Department of Agriculture Human Investigation Committee (Chairman), the U.S. Food and Drug Administration (FDA), U.S. Pharmacopoeia Convention, the National Institutes of Health (NIH), the World Health Organization, UNICEF, and the American Board of Internal Medicine. He has worked on international nutrition programs in several countries, including China, Guatemala, Haiti, Iran, Iraq, the Philippines, and Vietnam. Dr. Russell is a member of numerous professional societies, on the editorial boards of four professional journals, a past president of the American Society for Nutrition (ASN), and is now president of the ASN Foundation. Dr. Russell co-edited two editions of *Present Knowledge in Nutrition* and was the editor-in-chief of *Nutrition Reviews*. Dr. Russell served as a member of the National Academies of Sciences, Engineering, and Medicine (the National Academies) panels on Folate, Other B Vitamins, and Choline, and as chair of the panel on Micronutrients. He is a National Associate of the National Academies. He is former chair of the Food and Nutrition Board (FNB) of the National Academies, and is a fellow of ASN. Dr. Russell presently is working with the Biomarkers of Nutrition for Development (BOND) Program of NIH and is on the Board of Haiti Projects. He also has recently served as a board member of the Nestlé and Fetzer Foundations. He has received numerous national and international awards for his research on retinoids and carotenoids (Kritchevsky, Atwater, DSM awards), and has authored more than 300 scientific papers and 5 books. He received his M.D. from Columbia University.

Jamy Ard, M.D., is a professor in the Department of Epidemiology and Prevention and the Department of Medicine at Wake Forest University Baptist Medical Center. He is also co-director of the Wake Forest Baptist Health Weight Management Center, directing medical weight management programs. Dr. Ard received an M.D. and completed internal medicine residency training at Duke University Medical Center. He also received formal training in clinical research as a fellow at the Center for Health Services Research in Primary Care at the Durham Veterans Affairs Medical Center. Dr. Ard has more than 15 years of experience in clinical nutrition and obesity. Prior to joining the faculty at Wake Forest in 2012, Dr. Ard spent 9 years at the University of Alabama at Birmingham (UAB) where he served as medical director of UAB's EatRight Weight Management Services, vice chair for clinical care in the Department of Nutrition Sciences, and associate dean for clinical affairs in the School of Health Professions. Dr. Ard's research interests include clinical management of obesity and strategies to improve cardiometabolic risk using lifestyle modification. He has been conducting research on lifestyle modification since 1995 and has worked on several NIH-funded multicenter trials, including Dietary Approaches to Stop Hypertension (DASH), DASH-sodium, and Weight Loss Maintenance Trial. His work has been published in numerous scientific journals, and he has been a featured presenter at several conferences and workshops dealing with obesity. Dr. Ard has served on several expert panels and guideline development committees, including the Institute of Medicine Committee on Consequences of Sodium Reduction in Populations, the American Heart Association/American College of Cardiology/The Obesity Society Guideline Panel on the Identification, Evaluation, and Treatment of Overweight and Obesity in Adults, and currently, the American Psychological Association Obesity Guideline Development Panel. He is also serving on the editorial board for the *American Journal of Clinical Nutrition* and the *International Journal of Obesity*.

Stephanie A. Atkinson, Ph.D., D.Sc. (Hon.), is a professor and nutrition clinician-scientist, Department of Pediatrics, associate member, Department of Biochemistry and Biomedical Sciences, Faculty of Health Sciences, McMaster University, and professional staff in McMaster Children's Hospital, Hamilton. A key focus of her research has been investigations of the factors influencing skeletal development in premature and term infants and in children with bony morbidity secondary to disease process and/

or drug therapy (particularly steroids) in diseases such as lymphoblastic leukemia, nephrosis, rheumatoid disorders, cystic fibrosis, or epilepsy. Her current research encompasses clinical trial and epidemiological investigations of the environmental (nutrition), genetic, and biochemical factors during fetal, neonatal, and early childhood life that play a role in defining the offspring phenotype and as risk determinants for noncommunicable diseases. She leads a multidisciplinary team of researchers in the conduct of randomized clinical intervention trials of nutrition and exercise in pregnancy designed to optimize maternal and child health outcomes including bone health. Dr. Atkinson served on the Scientific Oversight Committee for the Dietary Reference Intakes (DRIs) from 1995 to 2004 and several DRI projects and workshops since that time, most recently as a working group member for the DRI and Chronic Diseases Endpoints project cosponsored by Health Canada and the Office of Dietary Supplements of NIH. Dr. Atkinson currently serves as chair of the Board of Directors of the Maternal, Infant, Child and Youth Health Research Network (MICYRN) and co-lead of the MICYRN Canadian Birth Cohort Coalition to harmonize data from Canadian birth cohort studies, as Executive Member of Board of Trustees of the North American International Life Sciences Institute (Washington, DC), and as a member of the Scientific Advisory Council for Osteoporosis Canada. Dr. Atkinson is an elected fellow of both the American Society for Nutrition and the Canadian Academy of Health Sciences and was recently awarded a Doctor of Science, honoris causa, from Western University in London, Canada.

Carol J. Boushey, Ph.D., M.P.H., R.D., is the director of the Nutrition Support Shared Resource at the University of Hawaii Cancer Center. Her research has involved working as part of multidisciplinary teams, which is crucial for providing support to the member investigators of the Cancer Center as they design and conduct studies that include the collection and analyses of dietary intake and other nutritional issues. She specializes in the broad spectrum of evaluating dietary exposures with an emphasis on use of technology and assessing diverse racial/ethnic groups. In collaboration with scientists in engineering at Purdue University, she created the Technology Assisted Dietary Assessment program that uses image analysis and visualization on small mobile devices (e.g., mobile telephones), to aid researchers to collect dietary intake with limited burden. She has been fundamental in describing dietary intakes of several Pacific Northwest Tribal Nations and young children in jurisdictions in the Pacific. Dr. Boushey is actively involved with the dietary assessment methods used with the Multiethnic Cohort (MEC), which includes 215,000 adults representing five ethnic groups (Japanese, Hawaiian, non-Hispanic white, African American, Hispanic/Latino). As a member of the Dietary

Patterns Methods Project, she completed analyses in the MEC showing that consuming a dietary pattern that achieves a high diet-quality index score is associated with lower risk of mortality from all causes, cardiovascular disease, and cancer in adult men and women. She has been the chief architect of paper- and computer-based dietary assessment methods to assess calcium consumption among Asian, Hispanic, and non-Hispanic white adolescents in the United States. Dr. Boushey received her Ph.D. from the University of Washington and her M.P.H. from the University of Hawaii at Manoa.

Susan M. Krebs-Smith, Ph.D., M.P.H., is the chief of the Risk Factor Assessment Branch of the Epidemiology and Genomics Research Program (EGRP) in the National Cancer Institute's Division of Cancer Control and Population Sciences (DCCPS). She oversees EGRP's research portfolio and initiatives that focus on the development, evaluation, and dissemination of high-quality risk factor metrics, methods, tools, technologies, and resources for use across the cancer research continuum, as well as the assessment of cancer-related risk factors in the population. Her own surveillance research has emphasized trends in intake of foods and nutrients, especially fruits and vegetables; food sources of nutrients; and factors associated with the intake of foods and/or nutrients, using data from the National Nutrition Monitoring and Related Research Program. Her contributions in the area of dietary assessment methodology have focused on developing methods to assess dietary patterns and the usual intake of foods. Her efforts in dietary guidance and food policy include quantifying potential future demand for food commodities based on population-wide adoption of the *Dietary Guidelines for Americans* and census projections. Dr. Krebs-Smith provided data analyses and consultation in support of the last several editions of the *Dietary Guidelines for Americans* and was a member of the Institute of Medicine's (IOM's) Committee to Develop a Framework for Assessing the Effects of the Food System. Prior to joining EGRP, Dr. Krebs-Smith was the chief of the Risk Factor Monitoring and Methods Branch in the Applied Research Program (now the Health Care Delivery Research Program), DCCPS. She received her Ph.D. from The Pennsylvania State University and her M.P.H. from the University of Minnesota.

Joseph Lau, M.D., is professor emeritus in the Center for Evidence Synthesis in Health within the School of Public Health at Brown University and was the co-director of the Agency for Healthcare Research and Quality (AHRQ) designated Evidence-based Practice Center (EPC) at Brown. Prior to Brown, he was a professor of medicine and professor of clinical and translational science at the Institute for Clinical Research and Health

Policy Studies at Tufts Medical Center. He directed the Tufts EPC from 1997 until 2012 and led the production of more than 80 evidence reports, technology assessments, and comparative effectiveness reviews under contract with the AHRQ. He has served as a member of an FDA advisory committee, and as a member of an Food and Agriculture Organization of the United Nations/World Health Organization workshop. He served as a member on two IOM committees including Framework to Evaluate the Safety of Dietary Supplements and Standards for Clinical Practice Guidelines. He received his M.D. from Tufts University School of Medicine and completed a fellowship in clinical decision making and medical computer science at the New England Medical Center.

Bruce Y. Lee, M.D., M.B.A., is an associate professor of international health at the Johns Hopkins Bloomberg School of Public Health, executive director of the Global Obesity Prevention Center (GOPC) at Johns Hopkins, and director of operations research at the International Vaccine Access Center (IVAC) as well as associate professor at the Johns Hopkins Carey Business School. Dr. Lee has more than 15 years of experience in industry and academia in systems science and developing and implementing mathematical and computational methods, models, and tools to assist decision making in public health and medicine. He has been the principal investigator for projects supported by a variety of organizations and agencies including the Bill & Melinda Gates Foundation, NIH, AHRQ, the Centers for Disease Control and Prevention (CDC), UNICEF, the Global Fund, and the U.S. Agency for International Development (USAID). His previous positions include serving as Senior Manager at Quintiles Transnational, working in biotechnology equity research at Montgomery Securities, and co-founding Integrigen, and serving as an associate professor at the University of Pittsburgh, where he founded PIHCOR (Public Health Computational and Operations Research), which is now based at Johns Hopkins. Dr. Lee has authored more than 180 scientific publications (including more than 90 first author and more than 35 last author) as well as 3 books: *Principles and Practice of Clinical Trial Medicine, What If . . .?: Survival Guide for Physicians*, and *Medical Notes: Clinical Medicine Pocket Guide*. He is an associate editor for the journal *Vaccine* and deputy editor for *PLOS Neglected Tropical Diseases*. He is a regular contributor to *The Huffington Post* and *Forbes*. He and his work have garnered attention in leading media outlets such as *The New York Times*, *Los Angeles Times*, *Time*, *CBS News*, *Businessweek*, *U.S. News & World Report*, *Bloomberg News*, *Reuters*, and National Public Radio (NPR). Dr. Lee received his B.A. from Harvard University, M.D. from Harvard Medical School, and M.B.A. from the Stanford Graduate School of Business. He completed his internal medicine residency training at the University of California, San Diego.

Joanne R. Lupton, Ph.D., is a distinguished professor emerita at Texas A&M University, where she was a faculty member for 31 years prior to retiring in 2015. She chaired the Macronutrients Panel for the Dietary Reference Intakes that determined the intake values for protein, carbohydrates, fats, fiber, and energy for the United States and Canada and she also chaired the IOM panel to determine the definition of dietary fiber. She was a member of the 2005 U.S. Dietary Guidelines Advisory Committee. She is currently serving a second term on FNB. Dr. Lupton spent 1 year at FDA helping to develop levels of scientific evidence required for health claims. While there she was appointed to the Commissioner's Task Force for Better Nutrition and received a Commissioner's Special Citation for her work. She was elected to the National Academy of Medicine in 2010 and is a lifetime associate of the National Academy of Sciences. Dr. Lupton has mentored more than 100 M.S. and Ph.D. students while at Texas A&M, and received the Dannon/ASN mentoring award in 2004. In 2007 she received the Texas A&M University distinguished achievement award for research. In 2010 she received the ASN General Mills Bell Institute of Health and Nutrition–Innovation Award. Dr. Lupton is past president of the ASN, the nutrition research organization. Her research is on the effect of diet on colon physiology and colon cancer with a particular focus on dietary fiber and n-3 fatty acids. She has received the Vahouny Medal for her research on dietary fiber. She translates basic research on diet and colon physiology to science-based public policy, and has consulted with individuals in China, Japan, South Korea, Taiwan, and elsewhere on the definition of dietary fiber and establishing dietary guidance systems in those countries. Her undergraduate degree is from Mt. Holyoke College and her Ph.D. in nutrition is from the University of California, Davis.

Sally C. Morton, Ph.D., is the dean of the College of Science at Virginia Tech, and holds the Lay Nam Chang Dean's Chair. Her research focuses on evidence synthesis and patient-centered comparative effectiveness research. Previously, Dr. Morton served as chair of the Department of Biostatistics in the Graduate School of Public Health and director of the Comparative Effectiveness Research Center at the University of Pittsburgh, vice president for statistics and epidemiology at RTI International, and head of the RAND Corporation Statistics Group. Dr. Morton was president of the American Statistical Association and chair of Section U (Statistics) of the American Association for the Advancement of Science, and she is a fellow of both organizations. She is a member of the Patient-Centered Outcomes Research Institute Methodology Committee, and the AHRQ EPC Program Methods Steering Committee. She has served on several National Academies committees, the Census Scientific Advisory

Committee, and the National Academies Committee on National Statistics. Dr. Morton holds a Ph.D. in statistics from Stanford University.

Nicolaas P. Pronk, Ph.D., is the president of the HealthPartners Institute and Chief Science Officer at HealthPartners and holds a faculty appointment as Adjunct Professor of Social and Behavioral Sciences at the Harvard T.H. Chan School of Public Health in Boston, Massachusetts. Dr. Pronk's work is focused on connecting evidence of effectiveness with the practical application of programs, practices, policies, and systems that measurably improve population health and well-being. His research interests include workplace health and safety, obesity, physical activity, and systems approaches to population health and well-being. Currently, Dr. Pronk serves as a co-chair of the U.S. Secretary of Health and Human Services' Advisory Committee on National Health Promotion and Disease Prevention Objectives for 2030 (Healthy People 2030) and is a member of the Community Preventive Services Task Force. He was the founding and past president of the International Association for Worksite Health Promotion and has served on boards and committees at the National Academies; the American Heart Association; and the Health Enhancement Research Organization, among others. He is widely published in both the scientific and practice literatures with more than 400 articles, books, and book chapters and is an international speaker on population health and health promotion. Dr. Pronk received his doctorate degree in exercise physiology at Texas A&M University and completed his postdoctoral studies in behavioral medicine at the University of Pittsburgh Medical Center at the Western Psychiatric Institute and Clinic in Pittsburgh, Pennsylvania.

Susan B. Roberts, Ph.D., is the director of the Energy Metabolism Laboratory, professor of nutrition and co-director of the Obesity Research Cluster in the Jean Mayer Human Nutrition Research Center on Aging at Tufts University, and professor of psychiatry and scientific staff member in pediatrics in the Tufts University School of Medicine. She received her Ph.D. from the University of Cambridge, United Kingdom, and did postdoctoral training at the Massachusetts Institute of Technology before moving to Tufts in 1987. Her research focuses on determinants of weight regulation, including dietary composition factors such as glycemic index, protein and fiber, and behavioral factors in weight control. In addition to her work in the United States she has conducted studies in the Brazil, China, The Gambia, Guinea Bissau, and the United Kingdom. She has published more than 240 research papers in research journals, including the *New England Journal of Medicine* and the *Journal of the American Medical Association*, and has an H-index of 61. Dr. Roberts was the 2009 awardee of the E.V. McCollum award of the ASN to recognize the creativity and importance of her work on weight regulation, and the 2016 W.O. Atwater Lecturer for important contributions to nutrition and health worldwide.

A. Catharine Ross, Ph.D., is a professor and the occupant of the Dorothy Foehr Huck Chair of Nutrition in the Department of Nutritional Sciences at The Pennsylvania State University. As a nutritional biochemist, Dr. Ross has studied cellular factors involved in the biosynthesis and transport of vitamin A molecules. Her focus has been on the interaction of cellular retinoid-binding proteins and enzymes that esterify retinol for transport, storage, and oxidation with the intent to link biochemical findings with nutritional studies to better understand how vitamin A homeostasis is regulated by dietary status and metabolic conditions. She also investigates the role of retinoids in immune function, principally antibody production. Dr. Ross has received numerous awards, including the Mead-Johnson Award and the Osborne and Mendel Award from the ASN. She is active within a range of professional societies, including the American Association of Immunologists, Sigma Xi, and the American Physiological Society, and has served on a number of committees for the ASN and the Federation of the American Societies for Experimental Biology. Dr. Ross is a fellow of the American Association for the Advancement of Science and a member of the National Academy of Sciences. She chaired the committee on Dietary Reference Intakes for Vitamin D and Calcium and served on the FNB panel on Micronutrients for the Dietary Reference Intakes, and the committee on Opportunities in the Nutrition of Food Sciences. Dr. Ross is also a member of FNB. Dr. Ross received her Ph.D. from Cornell University in biochemistry and molecular and cell biology.

Barbara O. Schneeman, Ph.D., served as the higher education coordinator for the U.S. Agency for International Development (USAID). In this role, Dr. Schneeman worked with the higher education community to improve awareness of USAID opportunities and increase engagement avenues for the agency. Previously she served as the director of the Office of Nutrition, Labeling, and Dietary Supplements at FDA from 2004 to 2013. In that position, she oversaw the development of policy and regulations for dietary supplements, labeling, food standards, infant formula, and medical foods and served as U.S. delegate to two Codex committees (Food Labeling and Nutrition and Foods for Special Dietary Uses). From 1976 to 2004, she was a member of the nutrition faculty at University of California, Davis, and is currently emeritus professor of nutrition. She has been a visiting scientist at University of California, San Francisco (UCSF), and Assistant Administrator for Nutrition in the Agricultural Research Service of USDA. Professional activities include participation in

Dietary Guidelines Advisory Committees (1990 and 1995) and the FNB of the National Academies, among others. She is recognized for her work on dietary fiber, gastrointestinal function, and policy development in the area of food and nutrition. She received her B.S. degree in food science from the University of California, Davis; her Ph.D. in nutrition from the University of California, Berkeley; and her postdoctoral training in gastrointestinal physiology at Children's Hospital in Oakland, California.

Martín J. Sepúlveda, M.D., FACP, FAAP, FACOEM, is an IBM fellow and elected member of the National Academy of Medicine. He is recently retired from the IBM Corporation where he had a distinguished career, serving in numerous executive capacities including vice president of Health Systems and Policy Research and vice president of Integrated Health Services. He led health policy, strategy, health benefits, services and operations, occupational health, and well-being for IBM globally. He is widely recognized for contributions in public and population health, private-sector health care, wellness, and health benefits innovation. He led private-sector collaboration with clinicians for medical home transformation leading to formation of the Patient-Centered Primary Care Collaborative. Dr. Sepúlveda received his M.D. and M.P.H. degrees from Harvard University, his B.A. magna cum laude from Yale University, and he completed residencies in internal medicine at UCSF Hospitals, and occupational/environmental medicine at the National Institute for Occupational Safety and Health. He trained in the Epidemic Intelligence Service of CDC, and completed a fellowship in internal medicine at the University of Iowa Hospitals and Clinics. He serves on several boards including the American Board of Internal Medicine Foundation, The New York Academy of Medicine, and the Council for Health Research for Economic Development.

STAFF

Samantha M. Chao is a senior program officer at the National Academies. Previously she was a manager at The Pew Charitable Trusts where she developed and implemented a process to ensure the integrity and quality of research produced by teams across almost 30 policy areas. In that role, she advised teams on design and conduct of high-quality research methods at the national, state, and local levels. At Pew she also worked on the State Health Care Spending project to enumerate the cost of health care to states. Prior to joining Pew, she directed numerous studies at the National Academies, including the groundbreaking report *Health IT and Patient Safety*. She focused primarily on health care quality; performance measures; payment models; and methods to improve the quality and value of health care through the strengthening of research, and also conducted studies related to the U.S. Social Security Administration; integrative medicine; and continuing education for health professionals. She completed an M.P.H. in health policy with a concentration in management at the University of Michigan.

Meghan E. Quirk is a senior program officer on FNB. Dr. Quirk's current projects include working with a committee to develop a workshop on federal, state, tribal, and local strategies to limit sugar-sweetened beverages among young children and assisting on a study to review the process for updating the *Dietary Guidelines for Americans*. Dr. Quirk has also worked on the recently completed review of the Special Supplemental Nutrition Program for Women, Infants, and Children (WIC) food packages and directed a study on interpreting reports on obesity prevalence and trends. Prior to joining the National Academies, Dr. Quirk was a postdoctoral research associate at Tennessee State University where she gained experience in community-based participatory research. She was part of a collaborative team that developed a smartphone app designed to provide nutrition education information to families with a preschool-aged child enrolled in WIC. She earned her doctorate from Emory University, where her research focused on the clinical and dietary evaluation of patients prescribed a newly approved drug for the management of phenylketonuria. During her graduate training, she was also involved in efforts to develop nutritional management guidelines of five inborn errors of metabolism. She earned her bachelor's degree in nutrition and dietetics from the University of New Mexico.

Anna Bury is a research associate at the National Academies. She is jointly supporting the consensus study that is reviewing the process to update the *Dietary Guidelines for Americans*, and the Food Forum, a longstanding initiative of FNB. During her time at the National Academies, she has assisted with two additional consensus studies, *Assessing Prevalence and Trends in Obesity: Navigating the Evidence* and *Finding a Path to Safety in Food Allergy: Assessment of the Global Burden, Causes, Prevention, Management, and Public Policy*. She received her bachelor's degree in public health and sustainable development from Gordon College, where her research focused on the relationship between sustainable agricultural systems and community health, with case studies in Morocco, Switzerland, and the United States.

Meredith J. Young joined FNB as a senior program assistant in September 2016. She is jointly supporting the consensus study that is reviewing the process to update the *Dietary Guidelines for Americans* and a workshop titled *Strategies to Limit Sugar-Sweetened Beverage Consumption in Young Children*. Prior to joining the National Academies, she worked at Virginia Polytechnic Institute and State University as a health education office assistant and an undergraduate research assistant. She has experience supporting clinical research, specifically controlled feeding studies assessing the effects of prebiotic supplementation and cocoa supplementation in pre-diabetic adults, the effects of high-sugar diets in children, and the effects of high-fat feeding in college-aged males. She received her bachelor's degree in human nutrition, foods, and exercise with a concentration in dietetics from Virginia Polytechnic Institute and State University.

Ann L. Yaktine is the director of FNB of the National Academies. The FNB applies scientific knowledge to advise the nation on policies related to food, nutrition, and food safety, and their roles in health maintenance and disease prevention. In her role as director, she is responsible for developing, implementing, and managing the board's activities, as well as engaging FNB members in strategic planning to identify important and emerging issues in nutrition and food sciences, and food safety. Dr. Yaktine is a 2008 recipient of the IOM's Cecil Award. In 2009 she participated in the Korea–U.S. Symposium on the Science of Food Safety Assessment. She has published journal reports on nutrition and cancer, nutrients and contaminants in foods, and nutrition assistance programs. Dr. Yaktine is a member of the Academy of Nutrition and Dietetics and the ASN. She holds an M.S. in nutrition from the University of Kansas and a Ph.D. in biochemistry and cancer biology from the Eppley Institute for Research in Cancer and Allied Diseases at the University of Nebraska Medical Center.

Appendix D

Disclosure of Conflicts of Interest

The conflict-of-interest policy of the National Academies of Sciences, Engineering, and Medicine (www.nationalacademies.org/coi) prohibits the appointment of an individual to a committee like the one that authored this Consensus Study Report if the individual has a conflict of interest that is relevant to the task to be performed. An exception to this prohibition is permitted only if the National Academies determine that the conflict is unavoidable and the conflict is promptly and publicly disclosed.

When the committee that authored this report was established a determination of whether there was a conflict of interest was made for each committee member given the individual's circumstances and the task being undertaken by the committee. A determination that an individual has a conflict of interest is not an assessment of that individual's actual behavior or character or ability to act objectively despite the conflicting interest.

Dr. Jamy Ard was determined to have a conflict of interest because in addition to his academic appointments, he serves as medical director for a medical food-based program that is owned by a company in the food industry.

Dr. Susan Roberts was determined to have a conflict of interest because she serves as chief scientific advisor and shareholder of a weight management company.

Dr. Barbara Schneeman was determined to have a conflict of interest because she serves on two scientific advisory councils in the food and agriculture industries.

In each case, the National Academies determined that the experience and expertise of the individuals were needed for the committee to accomplish the task for which it was established. The National Academies could not find other available individuals with the equivalent experience and expertise who did not have conflicts of interest. Therefore, the National Academies concluded that the conflicts were unavoidable and publicly disclosed them through the National Academies Current Projects System (www8.nationalacademies.org/cp).